To my God,

who eagerly offers His blessings when I
have no clue what the hell is going on.

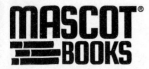

www.mascotbooks.com

Thank You Kung Fu

For more information, please contact:
Mascot Books
620 Herndon Parkway, Suite #320
Herndon, VA 20170
info@mascotbooks.com

Library of Congress Control Number: 2018901085

CPSIA Code: PBANG0418A
ISBN-13: 978-1-68401-504-7

Printed in the United States

THANK YOU
KUNG FU

David V. Wenzel

CONTENTS

PREFACE
THE HUT

THE SEIZURE HITS ME IN THE MIDDLE OF THE WOODS. I stumble, my right side having gone weak, and my knees hit the ground. I start to fall forward, but my right hand catches hold of a tree trunk just off the path. Everything is quiet. Crickets stopped chirping their evening songs, and the squawks of the local birds seem to have paused. Everything feels wet: my breath in the air, the ground on my knees, the bark on my hands. I feel my crotch to make sure I didn't piss my pants this time.

I know I need water, so I struggle to my feet and begin limping the hundred yards back toward The Hut. I stumble through the unlocked door and make sure not to lock it behind me in case someone, unfortunately, needs to come looking for me. I sit down on the bed. The right side of my body feels like Jell-O as I sip from my bottle containing reverse-osmosis water that was filtered twice before being alkalized to 9.5 pH to provide additional electrolytes. I can feel the drops leaking down the right side of my face, which has gone completely numb. I close my eyes, put one foot on the ground to stop the dizziness, then lean back onto my bed in my tiny cabin somewhere in the woods. My family is always concerned this will happen, concerned that when I go off on my own, I'll have a seizure alone in the dark and die by myself. But I had told them, "I can't live my life in fear that a sudden seizure will hold me back." And should a seizure be the cause of my early death in a tiny little hut, in the middle of a quiet forest, so be it. I really can't imagine a better way to go. Dust-to-dust and whatnot.

The day before, I had parked my car and began my walk for three days of complete solitude. I cry every single time I walk out to the cabin, named The Hut. I physically feel the worries shedding from my back every time, as an overwhelming peace pulls me deeper into the forest. It was dark when I arrived, but it didn't matter. I know my path through these woods. Take a hard right at the old barn. Slight left at the clearing. Slight right back into the trees and follow the winding trail to The Hut.

The Hut is small. There is no electricity or running water. It has a wood-burning stove and a single bed with flannel sheets. It has windows on all four walls, and there is a large painting of a grinning Amish farmer, who makes me wonder what he knows that I don't. There is a wooden porch out front with a two-person swing and a shed to keep the wood dry. The first thing I realize whenever I get to The Hut is how loud I am. Every noise I make is like a record scratch against the backdrop of silence. But eventually, my body realizes there is no hurry and I start slowing down my movements.

When I am at The Hut, I read, I write, I walk, and I nap. There are no other options. Through the purging of all distractions, I finally feel able to quiet the clutter in my head. I sit, accept the silence and, when I'm ready, let the words pour out of me. This is the place where a single day feels like three, and the accomplished work would agree.

Feeling steadier after my seizure in the woods, I undress for the night. I step outside to the ledge of the front porch, and, standing in my underwear and untied boots, I pee into the valley before me. When I'm nearly finished, I hear a pack of wolves, maybe a mile away, howling away at the bright full moon. My eyes widen as I start grinning from ear to ear. It seems quite obvious that I am part of their pack tonight. So, I do as any red-blooded boy would do and begin howling with them in the middle of our woods.

My howl is a celebration of surviving my previous five years with terminal brain cancer, after I was told I'd only have five to seven years left. With each howl, I burn through all of my frustrations, angers, and worries till I am gasping for breath.

And as I listen to my echo, I hear the short, eager yelps of the small pups, followed by the alpha male, crooning into the night with its deep voice. That last holy howl seems to be the final note to this choir of carnivorous beasts, each knowing its purpose in life: to eat, to breed, and report the news to the moon. It only lasts a few minutes, but those minutes are glorious for me. I hope they heard my howls and understand that I, like them, am a survivor.

I return inside, invigorated by that moment, and write by candlelight for a few hours before sleepiness sets in. I have no idea what time it is because, intentionally, there are no alarm clocks, no watches, and no phones. There is only sun or no sun. I tend the fire for the evening, prepping it for eight hours of warmth, and climb into bed.

I don't know how long I've slept, but when I wake up in the dark I can only hear the quiet. No humming of the refrigerator. No heat clicking on and off. No buzzing of electrical outlets. No distant car horns from across town. The only thing I can hear is a faint ringing in my ears. Eventually, I fall back to sleep and wake up to the sun.

While lying there with early morning sunlight peeking through the windows, I begin thinking through my King David complex. I feel God has put me on this earth to accomplish something I have not yet done. David was unafraid to face Goliath because he knew God wouldn't let him die before fulfilling His promise to make him king, and I realize I'm starting to hold God to a similar agreement. Until I do what He's created me to do, I must press forward with as little fear of death as possible.

I climb out of bed and returned to the ledge of the front porch to, well, you know, and I see footprints of a buck that had visited in the middle of the night to sniff my pee and determine my threat level. Not sure what his final decision was, but I feel worthy of being considered a threat. Maybe he was concerned a howling wolf had moved in the night before.

I had come to The Hut to write a speech. And when I return to the city, I'll be giving this speech at my five-year cancerversary party. We've invited nearly a hundred people to join us for dinner and drinks at a restaurant near Lake Michigan to celebrate surviving another year. But this year's cancerversary is unique. After surviving for five years, the cancer community declares you a "cancer survivor." But all I got from the American Cancer Society was a stock letter congratulating me on not dying, so I decided to throw my own party to properly celebrate.

In order to write this speech, I sit and scroll through my journals I've brought along to think through the absurdity of everything that has happened to me over the past five years. Five years of struggling to make enough money to eat, to pay rent, to repay debt, to save relationships, and to simply stay alive (both physically and metaphorically). While reading through them, I see so many interactions that hurt me so badly, namely with Amy. But in the end, I can't deny the fact I've been a miserable person as well. I know I have hurt others. So, in an effort to show respect and honor to those involved, I will only use my journals to recount the events that happened and not assume the feelings of anyone else involved, let alone convict them for their actions.

Now I write, attempting to downsize all of these massive moments into this tiny little speech; another cliché to toss into a world filled with problems way worse than mine. But please, understand I need this moment for myself. In the words of Josh Ritter, my favorite musician: *"Don't say it's been done a hundred thousand times cause this one is mine."* I know people have come before me, and I know people will come after me, but before anything else can happen, I have to get this story off my chest. It's been too hard to lug these word-filled chapters around with no one reading them.

When thinking through the words of my speech, I am motivated by a dream I had several years ago. The actual dream consisted of simple white text on a black background: "2 Corinthians 2:14." In fact, it wasn't as much a dream as it was a pointing finger. I suppose that's evidence I'm not very good at interpreting dreams. Apparently, God has to literally drop a reference—chapter and verse—on me. But being unfamiliar with this passage, I rolled over, grabbed my Bible, and looked it up.

> *But thanks be to God,*
>
> *who in Christ always leads us in triumphal procession*
>
> *and through us spreads the fragrance of the knowledge of him everywhere.*
>
> *For we are the aroma of Christ to God*
>
> *among those who are being saved*
>
> *and among those who are perishing,*

to one a fragrance from death to death,

to the other a fragrance from life to life.

Who is sufficient for these things?

For we are not, like so many, peddlers of God's word,

but as men of sincerity, as commissioned by God,

in the sight of God

we speak in Christ.

I feel shameful saying the aroma of my life has anything to do with Jesus Christ. I am far too aware of how bent I am. But Christ, through all my weaknesses, has made me sufficient. I can't even begin to determine how you will react to both the life and the death of my crazy existence. All I know is that my life will be an aroma of death to some—to those who refuse to believe the Spirit of God is active and working on behalf of us all, to those who believe I'm selfish or manipulative for sharing my story, to those choosing to ignore the stirrings in their hearts as they turn these pages. But I also know my life will be an aroma of life to others—to those who have placed their hope in the life, death, and resurrection of Jesus Christ, and to those willing to follow him through the pain and suffering this world offers. Above all, I hope I can share the main thing I've learned through my years of struggle, which I desperately hold onto every single day: *What God originates, He orchestrates.*

While finishing the writing of my speech, I notice a small newspaper article that had been cut out and pinned to the wall. It states that, two years ago, a devastating F4 tornado had torn through my pissing valley and came extremely close to demolishing my hut. Since the tornado had destroyed nearly all the trees in front of me, I can see through my window the destruction only a hundred yards ahead. Massive trees that had been standing for who knows how long had been shredded and ripped down. As I look back at the article, I notice a tiny Mennonite church business card pinned on the wall with a handwritten message:

The voice of the Lord breaks the cedars. The Lord breaks in pieces the cedars of Lebanon. He makes Lebanon leap like a calf, and Sirion like a young wild ox. The voice of the Lord twists the oaks, and strips the forest bare. And in His temple, all say, "Glory." (Psalm 29)

Sitting at my desk, I am forced to review the evidence that God can bring down a track of hundred-year old sinless trees and make them stay silent for a hundred more. This seeming train wreck against the act of creation, brought on by what seems like an angry God, is now home to new creatures who are telling new stories. And now, sitting here and writing about my own slowly rebuilding valley, I realize maybe He's done the same with me. God is a good God who creates, but God is also a good God who knows when to hit the restart button.

After the past years of my destruction, I now sit here as His destroyed but rebuilding temple, and I say *"Glory."*

ONE
TITS & ASS

"BUT WHAT ABOUT TITS AND ASS?" he yelled as he stood up, hushing the high school cafeteria around him. It was a bizarre question from a grown man to me, a sixteen-year-old student. Everyone's eyes widened as they looked at me and waited for my response.

"Well, we just…we can't. If we use those actual lyrics, we'll be disqualified. That's why we've changed it."

"You *changed* 'Tits and Ass'? To what?"

"We changed it to 'This and That'."

"'This and That'?" His volume increased as he realized he was now putting on his personal show, slightly grinning through his knowingly inane argument. "If you do that, you will defeat the actual purpose of the song! When that song was originally created, it blew everyone's mind. They were actually singing about what everyone else was only thinking. And now you've removed that powerful declaration of what 'Tits and Ass' actually meant to Broadway at that time. That song will completely lose its power if you choose to change those two words. Please, tell me who I need to talk to to change it back to 'Tits and Ass'!"

The guy saying this to me was Matthew Broderick. Yes, the Matthew Broderick you're thinking of. He was referencing the song, "Tits and Ass," from *A Chorus Line*, the musical I was currently practicing. My drama class, Play Pro, was nearly finished preparing our half-hour version of the show for the state finals. This conversation had begun in the cafeteria while having lunch, when Matthew asked me about my high school experience. I told him about playing in band and running track, but explained to him that practicing for *A Chorus Line* took the majority of my time. Being a stage actor himself, he got overly excited and asked if we were singing and dancing the original version of the 1975 Broadway play that was later recorded as a film in 1985 with Michael Douglas. I told him we were, which brought on the inevitable question, "But what about 'Tits and Ass'?" After my epic lunchroom reprimand, he asked if I would join him for breakfast at his trailer the next morning.

This entire scenario came about because I was selected for a speaking role in the movie *Election* that was being filmed at my school, Papillion La-Vista High School, in Papillion, Nebraska. I had auditioned, never dreaming I'd get the part and refusing to even get my hopes up. Then on October 15th, my sixteenth birthday, I received a call. I got the part. I would have a speaking role and share a few scenes with Matthew Broderick and Reese Witherspoon.

The first day I showed up on set, they took me to my trailer with my name and my character's name marked on the door: David Wenzel—Erik Overholdt. I'm surprised my grin fit through that door. I entered a perfectly clean trailer. I peed and flushed the toilet; it worked. I washed my hands in the sink; it worked. I tried the microwave; it worked. Then, left alone after trying the majority of major appliances, I sat on the couch for thirty more minutes having run out of things to do. The PA knocked on my door and took me to the makeup trailer. I was shocked when my makeup artist sat me in the middle of three seats. On the right sat Matthew Broderick and on the left sat Reese Witherspoon, each having their makeup done. I snuck a few peeks as they were putting a gruesome injury on Matthew's eye.

Next, they called me to the set. We filmed my scene three or four times and the director, Alexander Payne, who grew up in Omaha and typically filmed there, told me what a fantastic job I had done.

I get it: He probably tells this to all of the local first-time actors. But then he told me he wanted to make a last-minute change and expand my character to another role as well. This meant I would need to come back to film the next morning. *Perfect*, I thought. *I'll go to Matthew's trailer for breakfast, then go and complete this new scene.*

The next morning, I knocked on the door to Matthew's trailer. I was so nervous. He swung the door open and stood there, sans eye makeup, wearing a baggy t-shirt with boxers. He invited me in. I knew my career in Hollywood was quickly advancing when I realized his trailer was only slightly bigger than mine. He sat down to his breakfast while reading through our school newspaper. I smelled the coffee he'd just finished brewing. He asked if I wanted some cereal or perhaps a grapefruit. I wasn't sure I'd be able to eat it without throwing up all over his table, so I said no.

We sat across from each other as he engaged me in a pleasant conversation. I don't know why an A-list actor took any time at all to interact with a local teenage kid like me, but he actually seemed interested in me. With a big smile on his face, he asked me which of his movies was my favorite. I said *Glory*. He looked shocked, perhaps surprised to hear it wasn't *Ferris Bueller's Day Off*.

Eventually, the conversation ended up at *A Chorus Line* again. He laughed, still in shock from yesterday's news about changing the lyrics to one of the show's most famous songs. After a few more questions, he stopped and thought for a second. Sitting there, across from me in that slightly-bigger-than-mine trailer in his boxers and t-shirt, Matthew Broderick came to a conclusion. He settled into his seat, leaned back, squinted his eyes, and looked at me. It was as though he could see through my sugar-coated childhood when he said to me in a fatherly tone, "David, in this life you are going to have to choose between 'Tits and Ass' or 'This and That.' When these moments happen, I want you to make the right decision."

Trying to slow my heart rate after receiving a pep talk from Matthew Broderick, I simply uttered, "Okay."

I have never forgotten that moment because it felt like something inside of me changed. Looking back, it almost felt like that was the exact moment I moved from being a boy to being a man. Maybe I was drinking the Hollywood Kool-Aid, but for whatever reason, I actually believed him. I was old enough to see that everyone in my life was living a this-and-that existence. They didn't crave anything. But that wasn't me. I ached to travel. I was searching for incredible purpose. I yearned to be known for something. I desperately wanted people to be in awe of me. That life would be my tits-and-ass life.

Matthew's comment also brought back another memory to me, something strange that happened when I was ten years old. I remember being at my childhood home, 704 Edgewood Boulevard. Late one night, when I couldn't sleep, I was walking around the house, thinking thoughts far too big for my young brain. In the hallway upstairs, I saw the full-length mirror at the far end of it. I slowly approached it and looked at my young face. I tried to imagine what I would look like at twenty years, thirty years, even fifty years old. Strangely enough I couldn't see myself past fifty. It was as if my eyes couldn't manifest that image.

As I was looking directly at myself, I had an overwhelming feeling that my life would be used to accomplish something massive. That God had somehow made me to change other people's lives. And now, after Matthew's reminder, maybe it could be true that I was actually "set apart" and that I was made for so much more than This and That. Perhaps my life would carry such a unique purpose that people would need to hear about it, and if they didn't, they would be missing out on something important.

After that moment of standing and looking at myself in that mirror, my attitude changed and was rooted in the conviction that I was born a winner. I went into every situation determined to come out on top and to be the best and the brightest. From ten years old through high school graduation, I made up my mind to do extremely well in everything I set my hand to. Nothing was going to stop me from achieving even more of that success. And after my pep talk from Matthew Broderick, I was done settling for This and That. I wanted Tits and Ass.

In Fall 1999, I showed up to Cedarville University where I had been accepted. During my time at Cedarville, I met two people that would change my life forever. The first is Santino (Sonny) Stoner. He was a missionary kid from Spain whose family lived in Grand Rapids, Michigan. We developed a relationship based on our shared desire that media could truly change the way Christians thought about God. These years were the dawning of digital media, including music and movies. Napster had been created, and the university was completely clueless about the fact their students downloaded hundreds of pirated albums and movies. But Sonny and I were watching these films with different eyes. We both felt that film was never taken advantage of within the Christian community. Everyone was still trying to "reach" the lost people with clever sayings in little booklets of acrostics and simple line drawings. But Sonny and I were growing up in a new generation, and we were totally entranced by the media, the advertising, the music, and the films that surrounded us.

We were convinced that if we truly wanted to make a difference, it had to be through the best form of video, capable of competing with anything on MTV. We were tired of all the typical boring crap, never seeing any films of actual quality when it came to the Christian message. Caught up in this vision of what the future could be, we lay on the floor in my dorm room, praying that God would use us to do something, anything, to make a difference through film for our generation. Everything in the entire industry was This and That. And there, on the floor of my college dorm room, we felt called by God to introduce the Christian community to Tits and Ass. This moment was the beginning of something I never could have imagined at that time.

The second person to change my life was Amy, my future wife. She visited Cedarville my junior year, and I was completely smitten when I saw her. The first words she said to me were, "Do I look like a pimp?" (a comical reference to her outfit), and I knew then that I would marry her one day. After her graduation from Western Michigan University, she moved to Ohio to live with her sister for six months. It was so good to have her close. And soon, we determined that upon my upcoming graduation, we would both hit the road for Santa Monica, California, where she would live with her oldest sister, Angela. Amy said she always knew she would end up in California. I was happy to join her, knowing full well I could figure out a life for myself there.

It was a long drive we made, following each other in two packed cars. When we arrived, she fell on the floor in the middle of her sister's dark living room in pure exhaustion. I wanted to celebrate our arrival for the next portion of our lives together, so I snagged a bottle of vodka from the freezer and poured ourselves two shots. We clinked our glasses together, threw 'em back, and she passed out on the floor for the next several hours. Welcome to California.

We dated for three and a half years, and on July 23rd, 2005, Amy and I got married at the Round Barn Winery near St. Joseph, Michigan. Following our honeymoon to Puerto Vallarta, Amy got a job at an Outback Steakhouse and I worked at Famous Dave's. It was a wonderfully miserable time in our lives. Each night we'd come home, throw our tips onto the dresser, and compare our piles of cash as we shared stories of what happened that day. But our deep desires were still brewing in each of us. Amy started trying to put together photo shoots as I was trying to put together film shoots. We knew this is where we needed to be, and we were focused on what we were created to do.

Later I heard from a family friend that Trans World Radio, a global Christian radio organization, was looking for someone to make a series of short films describing the vast number of people around the world who were reached by radio every day. I contacted Barbara Shantz, the wonderful woman in charge of this project, and asked if I would be considered to take on that project. She confirmed they wanted to hire a director, but the decision would be made by the board who only met twice a year. I asked about the next time they would all be in the same room, and she told me it was for their yearly banquet at their headquarters in a few weeks. She told me the appropriate people needed to make a decision like this would all be there, but they wouldn't be able to have a meeting with me. Nevertheless, I told her I'd be there.

Of course it was a risk. But after my lesson from Mr. Broderick, I knew the worst thing that could happen was wasting $100 on gas to show up and simply ask. I packed the only suit I owned and drove thirteen hours to TWR's US headquarters in Cary, North Carolina, where my plan was to attend a meeting I was told couldn't be set up. When I arrived, I introduced myself to each of the board members, and they decided (I imagine out of sorrow for my trek) to have a quick meeting in a side room. I went in, pitched my concept, and upon returning home, learned I had won the work.

The TWR board told me to plan on shooting nine separate stories over five weeks in Europe, the Middle East, and Northern Africa. Amy expressed her concern with being left alone at home for five weeks, so I called Barbara and convinced her this project would be so much better if they had corresponding photography of the filmmaking process, as well as photos of the interview subjects, radio listeners, and scenery to use for their online and print marketing material. She agreed.

In 2006, Amy and I, along with a close friend serving as our cameraman, took off for five weeks to shoot in Ukraine, Austria, Albania, Slovakia, Italy, Poland, Jordan, and Morocco. We traveled everywhere, from Bratislava's medieval torture chambers (which apparently also served as inspiration for their similarly designed hotel rooms), to the rooftops of the incredibly designed Il Duomo Cathedral in Milan, to Jesus's rumored baptism spot just up the Jordan River from the Dead Sea, to a jailhouse cafeteria for lifelong prisoners in Wrocław, Poland, and to a tiny Moroccan village in the middle of the desert at the base of the Atlas Mountains.

One of my favorite memories of this trip was standing at the top of Mount Nebo, the resting place of Moses. To be standing there, where Moses stood, seeing the things that Moses saw, made me speechless. When you read about things like this in the Bible it's often difficult to imagine what it truly looked like, how it smelled, or the length of travel it so flippantly states. But now, standing on Mount Nebo, I was seeing the distance to the promised land. And being there in person, I could see it wasn't far at all. I could see the Jordan River directly below us as it ran into the Dead Sea. I could see on the map where Jericho used to stand and the small distances to Bethlehem, Jerusalem, and the Sea of Galilee. The Bible actually came to life right there in front of me as I took in what it must have been like for Moses to see the land that had been promised to His people by God. I was shocked at how quick the car trip was that took us down to the Jordan River, serving as the dividing line to Israel, God's chosen land for His people. Moses was so incredibly close to his home. But after spending forty years in the wilderness, fighting for and with his people, God proclaimed Moses would never enter that promised land. His marathon, his life, would end just before he crossed the finish line.

Previous to our trip, I had no idea how physically close he was when he laid down his head for the final time looking out over his people's promised land. Oh, to be so close to the thing you've been striving for for over forty years, yet be told it would never be yours. I couldn't possibly imagine what that must have been like for him. After all of those days lost in their journey, struggling, crying, and praying, the people were told by God that Moses died in peace, with "his eyes undimmed and his vigor unabated." It was there on Mount Nebo that I started to understand both the pain and pleasure conveyed by that famous quote by Havelock Ellis, "The only way to the promised land is through the wilderness."

This is a trip I never could have begun to imagine. I interviewed and filmed the stories of residents over three continents, sharing their life-changing messages, and seeing the world from the barren cliffs of Morocco to the top of historic cathedrals in Italy. Only three years after college, at twenty-four years old, I was a traveling filmmaker, married to a beautiful and brilliant photographer, sharing stories that actually mattered in order to change the world around me.

Tits and Ass, baby. Tits and Ass.

TWO
INSPIRATIONAL ARMS DEALER

THE ACCOLADES FOR MY TWR VIDEOS, as expected, never showed up. But to continue my career, I used them to get a job alongside Sonny.

Sonny introduced me to Brett VanTil, one of the producers of the NOOMA films, each of them a short sermon by Rob Bell filmed with incredible imagery and music. Brett was a hard-nosed businessman who owned a production company called Process that was doing great work for companies in Grand Rapids. On one trip to the West Coast, Sonny clicked with another individual, Corey Petrick, who said he stood for everything we did. Over the next two years, the four of us made constant progress to start a new production company called Dot&Cross. And in that time, we found another member, Gary Mahieu, who believed so deeply in what we did that he came on as a silent partner.

Over time we were able to work with people like Marcus Buckingham, Rob Bell, Francis Chan, Matthew Sleeth, Tim Keller, Josh Shipp, and Erik Wahl, and nonprofits like World Vision and Compassion International. Dot&Cross was making a difference! We were developing new and next-level products that were being ripped from the internet, while also being watched by presidents in the White House. Dot&Cross seemed like the work I was created to do. Not to act in Hollywood's films or be on Broadway's stage, but to help relay the messages of specific people, telling their stories to unite the public and make this world a better place. Yet still, despite our successful efforts, I was unable to find my own peace. I was creating with Dot&Cross while feeling the sharp sting of a rock in my own shoe, because I still wanted to tell my story. But my story didn't exist.

I suppose I was given a chance to truthfully create and tell my own story within my marriage. Amy and I were ridiculously similar. We were raised in strict Southern Baptist churches, and we connected through stories of our shared past experiences based in guilt. Both of us were looking for ways to branch out and cut ties with our pasts and former relationships. Amy was always more spiritually advanced than I was. I both loved and hated that about her. She didn't care about what anyone thought of her, while I stressed about other people's opinions constantly. She was always pursuing God, usually dragging me along behind her. We never ended up finding a church because Amy would call out something wrong about their theology or their practices at every one we visited. I wasn't nearly as concerned about the details as she was, but her refusal to attend gave me opportunities to sleep in or sit on the porch and journal over cups of coffee on Sunday mornings. I actually didn't mind at all.

Amy and I loved camping. We would go up north and climb the sand dunes, stop at a beach on the side of the road, and take hikes before we headed back to our tent at the Sleepy Bear Campground, passing honest campers (mainly RV-ers) who didn't leave their campsite for weeks or months at a time. We put together a set of camping gear based solely on my memories of once being a Boy Scout. But after a few of these trips, we agreed to make some changes. So, we traded in our sleeping mats for a queen-sized air mattress. We quit trying to make our own food and instead drove out to nearby restaurants. This type of camping was up both our alleys. After becoming an Eagle Scout in my teens, I no longer needed to prove anything regarding my camping skills. So, Amy and I decided to live the high-life of camping, or as it's recently come to be known, "glamping."

One weekend while we were up north, we realized they had shut down a lane on the Mackinaw Bridge that connected the upper and lower parts of Michigan. We saw there were masses of people walking across it, a tradition they do every Labor Day. We walked that four-mile bridge, an invisible line that that separates the lower peninsula from the upper peninsula and Lake Michigan from Lake Superior, in swimsuits and flip flops. People laughed at us for not thinking ahead, but who cares.

Amy was a terrific photographer. I would be in awe at the images she would bring home from each shoot. She always used light so perfectly in each photo. I often said, without even a hint of a lie, that she was the best children's photographer you could find. In fact, David Prince, head of BlackWater, hired Amy to come and photograph his family outside of Washington D.C. just weeks before he was called to sit in front of the Supreme Court to answer for the actions of his employees in the Middle East. I remember staring at his face on our TV screen and thinking to myself: *I sat on his porch and shared a beer with that dude two weeks ago.*

Eventually, I came to realize that Amy and I seemed to be fire and ice. On some days, we would be so in sync with each other, so in love with each other, that our creative minds would collaborate not only on work but also within each other's daily practices. And on other days, and often for no reason, we would be frigid to each other. Unfortunately, as our artistic pendulums swung back and forth, there were rarely times spent in the middle. I found that our marriage was, as Dickens said, "the best of times and the worst of times." But I knew the person I married and was entirely aware of this difference in us, yet I still desired to be with her.

There was one photographer Amy loved the most: Jasmine Star. And after a year or two it became quite obvious they were stalking each other online. So, on one of our trips to Los Angeles, Amy invited Jasmine to come up from Irvine so we could all meet up at Amy's cousin Todd's house. She was incredibly excited to meet another photographer of the same caliber whom she respected so much. I remember the doorbell ringing as I opened it to find Jasmine standing there. Even I had learned enough about her to be equally excited. And later, I was so pleased to meet her husband, J.D. We continued to hang out on that trip, but Amy and Jasmine became fast friends. Every time we went to L.A., we always made plans to spend time with them, eating, laughing, and telling stories about "the photography world." We would visit fancy restaurants, but the Stars were so remarkably generous they always went out of their way to pay for our meal, despite my best efforts to stop them. I even tried to offer our server my credit card halfway through the meal, but learned that J.D. had done the same thing when we walked through the front doors.

Everything in our lives seemed to be making progress. We were attempting to grow in our marriage, developing friendships with other couples like Jasmine and J.D. And I was attempting to grow in my position with Dot&Cross, which had become a smashing success. But it didn't feel like success for me. I was lost in the middle of it all, continually working while feeling no love for our projects. I stopped caring about those who watched the films we created. To me, it just turned into another job. I wasn't the only one. Somewhere in the middle of our company's growth, we all started making films to pay the bills and not because these messages desperately needed to be heard. We started upping our costs and downsizing our personal commitments to the final product. We had managed to ruin something beautiful.

We got greedy with our success. As the Content Architect for Dot&Cross, the first question I asked any new project moved from, "How are you going to change the world with this project?" to "Who is going to pay for this project?" The company ended up getting into fuzzy arguments with ourselves and our clients over dollars and royalties and ownership. In fact, right before the company started its decline, we experienced internal combustion between our partners. We turned down a $15 million project based on the "idea" we could get more for it somewhere else. It was at this point it became obvious we were looking for products not based in truth but market potential. I suppose it makes sense, right? That's how you move a business forward, but in the end, all you end up with is a successful business, whether or not the world has been changed. And showing up to work every day for a company like this turned out to be simply This and That.

I remember living in California years earlier and stopping in at the Santa Monica Promenade mall and coming across a book called *Blue Like Jazz* by Donald Miller. I sat down to read it and never got up. I called into work to tell them I was sick so that I could sit and read that entire book again the next day. This Donald Miller seemed like such a unique person. I remember dreaming that someday I could meet him and tell him how his honest look at faith had changed me.

Through Dot&Cross connections, we ended up in Don's third floor condo in Sellwood, Oregon. We had partnered with him to develop and write a ten-part TV series called *Transitus*, a term relating to passing through or transitioning. The best budget we were offered from a high-level publisher was $1 million dollars for the show's creation, but true to our new, more cynical natures, Dot&Cross determined we needed more money, so we passed. But through this process, I met Don and we remained close friends.

We visited Portland several times, and on one trip, he told us about this freak connection he made while speaking at a camp in British Columbia, Canada. It was a cold and rainy day, but Don and his friends decided to kayak up the Princess Louisa Inlet. Realizing how wet they were, and that the storm was worsening, they agreed they had made a mistake and started to turn around. Next, they looked over to see this large man running down to the water and waving them into his dock. They paddled their kayaks to him and got out to meet this giant man who was grinning from ear to ear. He called to his wife, who came out holding what looked like freshly baked chocolate chip cookies, and he gave Donald a big hug. "Hi, I'm Bob Goff," he said.

We were shocked as Don explained to us how he and Bob had developed a unique relationship. Bob asked Don what the best use for his massive cabin would be, and they agreed it would be a great place for creatives to get away, turn off their cell phones, and exist without computers or equipment. To simply exist for a few days in one of the most beautiful inlets in the world. So, Don and Bob invited Dot&Cross to the first Malibu Lodge Gathering in the summer of 2008.

At that time, I was taking flying lessons, so our pilot in Seattle offered me the chance to take off and fly over parts of the gorgeous Cascade Mountains during our one-hour flight to Malibu Lodge. As our plane crested over the final mountain, the pilot pointed out Bob's place. A massive log cabin, built forty feet above the inlet below. We circled the house before we came down to land our Beaver Seaplane in the inlet by the dock. Bob and his wife, Sweet Maria, hugged each and every person getting off the plane. This is how they greeted everyone who came to the lodge. And then, they went on to treat us like kings over the following few days. We ate together, talked together, cried together, and took the boat to local waterfalls and beaches together.

I remember when Bob put us all in a boat and took us up into the inlet. He dropped each one of us off in the middle of nowhere and said, "We'll be back in an hour!" We were able to spend time by ourselves in the absolute middle of the Canadian wilderness. Then back at the house, we played bocce ball, put together puzzles, and lined up to leap off a thirty-five-foot cliff into the inlet. That night we heard the roaring thunder rip through the blackest of nights as we all went outside to jump into the bioluminescent water, which glowed with every move we made. At night I shared a bunk bed with Stephen Opperman (the Heritage furniture designer), and our third roommate was the lead guitar player for Jars of Clay. The list of people that came to this event sent our company into shock. The visitors included musicians, filmmakers, writers, political figures, artists, and so on. And each of them were there for the same reason: to be recharged in order to keep fighting the good fight.

It was amazing to see how Bob interacted with this lodge family. He simply loved people. Merely hours after meeting him, he had somehow convinced me that he even loved me. No matter what I had created, no matter the quality of the content, no matter the reviews I received, or the payments I was given, I was loved by Bob.

As we met in the main house every day, Bob was revving us up to leave the lodge with our hearts full of love and return home to spill that love over everyone around us. No matter what project, no matter what payments, no matter what intent, Bob encouraged us to openly and freely share our love with others. We were given the compelling order to return home with nothing but love for ourselves, love for our families, love for our work, and love for those around us. It was, as Bob reminded us, what Jesus was best known for.

When we had to leave, the sea plane lifted us up out of the waters to take us back to Lake Washington in Seattle. We did a full U-turn before we flew back past the house at a low altitude. I watched as the entire Goff family, even Sweet Maria, jumped into the water with all of their clothes on. It was their personal family tradition; a caper to show their deep appreciation for our visit. I will never forget this moment. These few days, I knew, would change my life forever. It reinvigorated my desires to love my wife, love my family, and find unique ways to show my clients my love for them.

But over the next year, the cold bioluminescent water of the Princess Louisa Inlet that lit up my soul had dried up. The warmth from those late-night campfires had fizzled out, leaving me shivering around its ashes. And the thrill of leaping from thirty-five feet in the air could be easily mistaken for leaping off a building. I found myself in a marriage where conversations always seemed to end in arguments and moments shared together seemed to end in either numbness or bitterness. And each day I would enter into the bickering that plagued our company.

The next year, I made myself scarce at the office, setting up shop at the recently built Grand Rapids Art Museum or in the public park down the road. Working at our office on Ionia Avenue had turned into a nightmare. Every noise invaded my brain like a surprise terrorist attack. Every knock on the door, tapping foot, computer blip, sounded like a fire alarm inside my head. Either something was wrong with the world around me or something was wrong with me.

In the beginning of May 2009, the middle of my personal desert and end of my waning hope, I started avoiding the morning office hours by "concepting" at my favorite coffee shop, The Sparrows Coffee, Tea, and Newsstand. I would arrive at this quaint Parisian style café, order a coffee, and take a seat next to the back window where I always sat. I'll always remember the first time I sat there, noticing the spider webs haunting the tops of windows as if recently placed there by the art department. The café's music always served as the perfect soundtrack to that day's writing. But one morning, as I was working on an upcoming project, I was listening to my own music. Arcade Fire, one of my favorite bands, came on to serve as the pulse to which I would create.

As I listened to the final track on the Neon Bible album, entitled "My Body is a Cage," something strange happened. In the middle of my writing, I noticed the words in a completely different way than I ever had before. I knew the words but had never actually *listened* to them. But now I realized how familiar they sounded, because they perfectly described the nature of my life:

I'm standing on a stage

Of fear and self-doubt

It's a hollow play

But they'll clap anyway

I'm living in an age

That calls darkness light

Though my language is dead

Still the shapes fill my head

I'm living in an age

That screams my name at night

But when I get to the doorway

There's no one in sight

Those words were me. Those words cut to the core of what I was feeling, slicing my heart open to show me who I had finally become. I had lost my desire to create, to share, to preach what I believe. I had become another robot, simply showing up so I could get paid. And on top of that, my marriage to Amy was struggling. We were both moving forward, but it seemed like we were veering off in opposite directions. It seemed everything—my job, marriage, spirituality, and overall purpose—were caught in the lyrics of this song, whose verses were separated by this haunting chorus:

My body is a cage that keeps me

From dancing with the one I love

But my mind holds the key

There, sitting in this coffee shop off Wealthy Street, I lost it. Still early in the morning, I was the only person in the shop. I couldn't control what was happening to my body. My eyes started crying and my nose started running. And while attempting to stop this overwhelming mess, my body actually started shaking. I didn't look up, I was unable to look up, so I stared at my computer screen to avoid making eye contact with the owner who was serving coffee behind the bar. And despite this overwhelming breakdown of my body, my finger went back to replay the song again as my emotions kept sweeping over me. There was no way I could stop the tears from flowing. My breath stopped. My lips pressed together. My body shivered. My insides were clenched. On the verge of vomiting, I kept searching myself for some type of response. *Am I having a nervous breakdown? Am I having a panic attack? What is going on!*

I felt broken. My marriage and my career were all mangled up. I was alone on a stage, playing a hollow game, speaking a dead language, taking what I'd been given, living in an age that screams my name at night, and opening the door to see no one in sight. I felt the connection between my heart and my head was hijacked, and it hurt so badly not knowing what to do next. Now my body was attempting to bring this moment to my full attention. I felt like Moses. I saw the promised land—the perfect wife, the perfect job, the perfect friends—but somehow felt I would end up eternally stuck in the wilderness.

THREE
FUCK EXPERTS

"FUCK EXPERTS!" This choice of words may not have necessarily been the best, considering it was roared out in front of a room filled with four hundred individuals who paid good money to sign up and travel across the country to attend the "Experts" Academy. But this was Tony Robbins talking, and he was in the zone. The Experts in the room were taken aback at such a blatant affront, but I perked up and moved closer to the edge of my seat.

My business partner, Brett, and I had landed in San Francisco to attend Brendon Burchard's Expert Academy, a three-day conference at the Sofitel hotel, that promised to provide the tools necessary to become an expert in your particular field. I was unsure about going but hadn't been to San Francisco in several years and wanted to see it again. Plus, Michigan was making me tired. I was in a rut, working on projects I didn't care about so I could pay the bills, which in turn allowed me to work on more projects that I didn't care about. Something had to change.

At the beginning of the conference, Brendon told us how to greet each other over the next three days. When we met a stranger we should ask, "What are you an expert in?" It would be a great way to get to know why these people were in attendance. So, I would ask and they would say, "I'm a Pilates expert!" or "I'm a weightlifting expert!" Then I would say, "I am an expert in training other experts!" which always begged for further explanation. "Well," I'd say, "I am an expert in training other experts to communicate their message by creating films, writing books, marketing, and blogging on their behalf." That just confused people further. Halfway through day two I gave up trying to explain.

My new plan was to look people directly in the eye and tell them I was a kung fu expert. At least then I could enjoy them trying to process my response. I took far too much pleasure in watching people try to figure out whether I was being serious or not.

It was a struggle for me to sit through session after session of Brendon going on and on about how "Experts" are changing the game of business today. He discussed how to write efficiently for the web, how to create book proposals, how to market ourselves online, how to behave in interviews. For the most part it was a good conference, but I was so done with this type of thinking. I hated the fact people paid money to be trained on how to scam the system by declaring themselves experts. Near the end of the second day, he summed up his overall concept on how to become a certified expert in these three points:

First, know tons of information. This part is simple. By reading the right books and doing online research, it is possible to have "head knowledge" of just about anything in less than a month. Sure, you can't perform brain surgery, but you would know so much information you could easily breeze through intense conversations about brain surgery, or for that matter, landing on the moon, or disarming nuclear bombs.

Second, stand behind the information. If someone argues with you on the facts, simply deny it. Always. The internet has made so much information available regarding any statistic or research that you can take just about any view on any issue and find someone, somewhere who will back you up.

Third (and the most interesting), *take a unique, controversial stance on the issue.* Now, you must present your information through a different approach. This new approach is your level of differentiation that separates you from the other experts in the same field. And those who know very little about your field will think you are smart because you are rebelling against the way others in your field are thinking. In a room full of ninety-nine black shirts, we'll always find and focus on that single red shirt.

And then, in Brendon's personal *coup de gras*, he brought on, as a surprise to everyone in the room, Tony Robbins. If you aren't familiar with Tony, his physical presence is remarkable. He looks like Andre the Giant from *The Princess Bride,* and he actually pounds on his chest while he talks. Furthermore, and I kid you not, has a musical soundtrack that bubbles up as he starts harping on about a specific point. Then, as his voice lowers, the soundtrack does the same. I felt like standing up and asking if anyone else had just heard the *Braveheart* soundtrack like I just did.

But Tony was, technically, the best Expert in the room. First, he knew his information. Second, he stood behind his information. And, third, after taking two purposeful steps toward the edge of the stage, he ended his rant by shouting, "FUCK EXPERTS!"

We have four hundred Experts in a single room who showed up to hear Tony Robbins tell them to get fucked.

Tony yelled at us, asking if any of us had read a book focused on our respective industries. The number of hands raised was surprisingly low. He questioned us about the number of blogs pertinent to our expertise we read each day. Again, a surprisingly low number of hands went up. He screamed that if he had one month in a room with an espresso machine and a clear Wi-Fi signal, he could pummel each of us in our own field of expertise. He would be able to understand any industry, any sport, any hobby, any religion, and bury us in arguments regarding our own individual areas of expertise. In fact, he said it with such overwhelming force that even I believed him.

"But," he declared, easing off his attack position, "what I cannot take away from you is your experience, your scars, and the emotions you've felt. These are the things that separate you from anyone else who is scratching to get into your field of work. In this race we call life, truly winning has nothing to do with being an Expert. It has everything to do with being an Authority. Experts are in the middle of their sprint, while Authorities are struggling, only half way through their marathon. Being an Authority on an issue is entirely different from being an Expert. Experts talk a good game, like an announcer at a baseball game, but Authorities are the pitchers, standing on the mound, sweating it out in the bottom of the ninth inning. Same game; different roles. Experts know because they've read the article, but authorities know because they wrote that article. Same article; different roles. Authorities have gathered their research with their blood, their sweat, and their tears. They speak not with information but with wisdom. This is the problem with the world today: Everyone's an Expert, but no one is stepping forward to prove themselves as an Authority."

A brilliant light from heaven shone down upon my cherubic face. This is it; this is the truth. This difference between Experts and Authorities, was the Tits and Ass explanation I had been desperately searching for. Tony explained the hypocrisy I see between everyday businesses and the creative geniuses we rarely see. Experts are too focused on reporting their successes in the right places and at the right times. They know the right information and acquire the statistical knowledge to defend their information. But an Authority doesn't need to defend anything. There is no need to defend the memories you own or the emotions you've felt. And with this position of authority, comes confidence. This confidence is not based on successes, even though there have been many; it has been molded, built plank by plank, through the Authority's repeated failures.

I stumbled out of that room, holding back tears. The day was over, and I needed to be in a safe place. I called my friend, Josh Shipp, to ask if he could meet me. I boarded the next train to San Jose and one hour later arrived at Josh's house. Josh could tell something was wrong, so he left the family at home while we walked down to Crema coffee shop. We ordered and sat outside at a patio table. I tried to hold myself together but couldn't. Tears started flowing as I expressed my deep hurt. I had felt from a young age that I was created to do something different, to be "set apart." But it seemed I had only turned out to be a patsy, sharing the messages of other people around me. Josh understood. He knew all about this, having his own unique story of his own childhood pain.

How on earth could I be jealous of his childhood pain? I had no story to share. I had no unique experience I had to overcome. Jokingly, I told Josh a story of when I was three years old. I remember a very young boy, maybe eight years old, who started mowing the backyard of the babysitter's house where I was staying. I was standing there while he mowed the edge of the grass next to me. Suddenly, I got scared and attempted to turn around and run, but I fell over in front of the lawn mower. The mower blade went across the top of my left forearm, taking off a chunk of skin down to the bone. I remember looking down to see my bloody arm and going into shock. I still have a nasty scar, but at least I didn't lose the arm. I told Josh that I would be a different person if that lawnmower had actually taken my arm off; I would have my story of a struggle that I overcame. We started laughing about volunteering an arm for the sake of a personal purpose. But when the chuckles quieted down, I realized that maybe that life would have been better for me.

At the end of my frustrating visit with Josh, I told him a few of the lines from one of my favorite Morrissey songs that had been circling my head for months on end and had come into fruition on this very night:

Jesus hurt me when he deserted me,

but I have forgiven Jesus for all the desire he placed in me

when there's nothing I can do with this desire.

Why did you give me so much love in a loveless world,

when there's no one I can turn to to unlock all this love?

Why did you stick me in self-deprecating bones and skin, Jesus?

Do you hate me?

When I got back to the hotel, I got a drink at the bar with Brett and some other Experts. Each of us went around in a circle declaring what our expertise was in, and, of course, I told them I was an expert in kung fu. The guy next to me, who probably had too much to drink, was astonished by this news. He asked me to display some of my moves. Never one to turn down a moment like this, I started pulling out the minimal amount of moves I learned from watching *The Karate Kid*. They said I looked more like I was dancing, so when my instigator got up to show me his moves, we ended up battling each other in this overly dramatic dancing style of kung fu.

He did a roundhouse kick, and pretending he'd hit me in the face, I dramatically turned around and accidentally hit my head on a concrete pillar behind me. My hands immediately went to my head, making sure I wasn't bleeding. It didn't hurt, but I hung up my kung fu career at that moment. I turned back and smiled as I sat down. Everyone was laughing. My kung fu instigator settled in and asked me where I was from. I went to say Grand Rapids, but realized those words weren't exiting my mouth.

My hands shot up to my mouth, feeling my lips, my throat. Then to my head where I only had a small scratch. *Come on, David! Say it! Say, "Grand Rapids."* But I couldn't. I held up my hand and gave a nervous smile as I tried to calculate what was actually going on in my body. This had never happened before. I tried to force air out of my mouth, but with it came a shaky moan. I guess my eyes starting showing shock. The person I was talking to leaned in, "Are you okay, man?" My shaky smile returned, and I nodded my head. I closed my eyes and focused on my lips, trying to move them, but nothing would come out. My thinking was entirely clear, and I was internally yelling, *Talk! Say something!* My brain was shouting but my mouth was on mute.

I had garnered the attention of about six people around me who were now leaning in closer to show their honest concern. Now, I attempted to keep my cool with a plastic smile, but I was holding back a panic attack. I needed to get out. I couldn't handle all of these eyes looking at me without the ability to perform for them. I stood up, ready to bolt for the elevator when someone grabbed me, "Hold on!" they said, "You might have a concussion!" I gave them the look as if that was the craziest idea I'd ever heard. How would I know? I had never had a concussion before. All I knew is that I wanted to get out of there.

Brett, realizing the weight of this situation, leaned in and put his arm around me and whispered, "David, calm down. Can you say anything?" The tears were filling my eyes as I focused everything I had on my lips. I closed my eyes as tight as I could and tried to say something, "Pi-ll-ows." I looked at Brett, who heard it and gave a slight chuckle. "Ok, good!" Having heard myself speak, I tried again, "Con-c-crete." I had no idea where these words were coming from.

I started by focusing on my lips, attempting to put a small sentence together. "Hit muh hed." They all looked at me nodding their heads. I pointed upstairs, saying, "bed" and started to walk there. I suppose the crowd felt a little better about me talking, and they let me leave. While walking away, tears began flowing down my face. *What on earth is happening to me?*

I got to my hotel room as my voice was starting to return. I stood in front of the bathroom mirror looking at myself, "Dot un Coss, Grnd Raps, Mchgun, Hotl, A, B, D, 1, 3, 4." I could see the fear in my eyes as these words formed then fell out of my mouth. I sat on the bed, not sure what to do next. I had to talk to Amy. I waited until my voice sounded secure enough to talk normally. It was about 4:00 a.m. EST, but I had to call her. (Later after listening to the message at home, I was shocked to hear how strange I sounded.) I closed my eyes and tried to slowly put together sentences, but my speech was thick with obvious flaws. I lay down and, surprisingly enough, fell asleep quickly.

I woke up in the morning and went into the bathroom. Time to try again. "My name is David Wenzel. I am married to Amy and we live in Grand Rapids. I am a creative for Dot&Cross. I am in San Francisco." Huh. Everything was back to normal. Phew! I wasn't sure what had happened last night, but it had scared the crap out of me. I was about an hour out from the start of the last day of the conference, so I hopped in the shower.

Midway through my shower, I felt a weak tingling down the right side of my body. I grabbed the side of the tub. The feeling was much stronger than it had been the previous night. Again, I couldn't speak, but I also was having trouble holding myself up with my right arm. Then I started to taste metal in my mouth. As soon as that happened, I started spitting tons of saliva out of my mouth. I tried to talk, but only vacant moans came out. I began to panic but then realized small words were starting to come out of my mouth, and slowly they became clearer and clearer.

I immediately turned off the shower, grabbed a towel, and went to the mirror. "I am David Wenzel. I'm from Michigan. I'm married to Amy and work for Dot&Cross." Then I started moving my mouth as much as I could, doing wide stretches, then pursing my lips. It seemed like everything was working right now. Strange.

That moment was much worse than the incident from the night before. I was worried but thought that giving it additional credibility in my mind would only make the situation worse, so I again brushed it off. I sneaked in before the start of that first session and sat next to one of the friends I had met at the conference, Thomas Mai, the film festival expert.

Five minutes into that first session, my body started to get hot. I looked around, curious if anyone else was pulling at their collar. Had the temperature gone up? I undid another button and took a long draft from my water bottle, but I was still getting hotter and weaker. I felt like I was waking up from a deep afternoon nap under a hot down blanket. I was so tired, my ears started burning, and I was seeing tunnel vision. I could hear Brendon, but his words seemed to be coming out in slow motion. My body was shutting down. In an attempt to show resiliency, I leaned forward and tried to reach for my coffee on the table, but as I did so, I fell off my seat and passed out.

Passing out sounds scary, but it's not. It's that glorious feeling of finally falling asleep after hours and hours of trying to fight it, like in church or the classroom. It felt so peaceful. But more was happening to me than just unconsciousness. When I hit the floor, I suffered a grand mal seizure. My body started convulsing, muscles contracting and pulling against their opposing muscles, neck in full tension, teeth and toes fully clenched. I shook uncontrollably for five minutes. There was nothing anyone could do but sit and watch as my body went through this hell. At the end of those five minutes, my body rebooted, meaning I completely passed out for the next half hour as my body began to recover.

Years later, Brett told me that Brendon Burchard had recorded that whole conference. I hesitantly chose to watch it again. At that moment on the final day, with the video camera focused on him, you saw him stop talking. He peered toward the back of the room, and as the viewer, you could sense the hairs on the back of his neck standing straight up. Fear moved through his face as his Expert mask was cracked wide open. You could sense his noticeable tension. Everyone in that room turned in their seats as they began hearing the noises of metal chairs smacking together and yelling voices. And despite the fact I'm going through a seizure, you hear me cry out. In major seizures, muscles contract around the lungs causing them to close, pushing air up through the larynx. In the middle of all this commotion you hear my voice moaning, like the hauntings of a ghost, making its way up through my octaves of agony.

Later I saw that Brendon had posted this same video to his site and explained what to do when someone has a medical emergency in the middle of a session. I suppose it's what any refined Expert would have done in this situation; use someone's pain to show off his advanced expertise. But after watching this video, which focused on a life-changing moment for my future that seemed to be played off as a promotion for his next breakthrough conference, I was filled with rage. I couldn't help but agree with Tony: Fuck Experts.

FOUR
OPERATION 55 ZEBRA

FLIP FLOPS. They were the first thing I saw when I woke up. I followed the legs upward and realized it was Brett, still in his pajamas, standing in the middle of the parking lot. The open-mouthed, shocked look on his face told me everything. I was loaded and strapped into the ambulance by paramedics before they closed the doors and sped toward Stanford Hospital. My paramedic was holding my hand as I continued to regain consciousness and began to speak. The first thing I mumbled was, "What happened?" She explained that I had a grand mal seizure. I looked down, doing my personal analysis to see if anything was broken or missing. I saw my wristband. It was labeled, "Fifty-Five Zebra." "What's this?" I asked. She responded, "When we picked you up, we didn't know your name so our computer assigned you with call sign, Fifty-Five Zebra."

Strangely enough, I was actually feeling quite normal. Then I got embarrassed, thinking about how I'd been shaking uncontrollably in a room full of four hundred Experts. I asked her again, "I was on the ground shaking in front of all those people?" My paramedic confirmed it and explained a few of the people in the crowd were medical professionals (Experts, if you will) and alerted everybody about what to do. She asked me what happened, and I told her I hit my head on the concrete pillar in the lobby of the hotel the night before and had some problems talking. Then I explained the incident in the shower (less than two hours previously) where I couldn't talk and tasted metal. She told me it was most likely blood on the brain, which can cause seizures.

When we arrived at Stanford Hospital, my stretcher was removed from the ambulance and I was taken inside. I was feeling so awkward that all of these people in scrubs and doctors' coats were all focused on me. I needed to distract them by playing some jokes. Brett had followed us to the hospital and handed me my phone. I briefly called Amy to let her know I had passed out, but then I saw Brett had sent me a picture of me in my hospital gown on the stretcher. So, I tweeted about my situation and included the photo of me on the stretcher. There were several nurses who thought I was hilarious for tweeting about what was going on. I had the whole room in stitches. Humor: That's my go-to plan whenever I need to cover up how scared I feel.

They took me to my own room in the Intensive Care Unit. I felt so silly that I was in the ICU because I was feeling fine. A few doctors came into the room and asked me to repeat the story of hitting my head the night before and of my incident in the shower. Each story was followed up with me saying, "But I feel fine now!" Nevertheless, they had to perform a CAT scan, x-rays, and an MRI. This was my first time in an MRI machine. I'd seen enough episodes of *House* to know they were extremely loud.

I was sitting in my ICU room with Corey, a nurse who was only a few years older than me. More lab coats came in to ask a few more questions. Then a woman came in and told me she was my actual doctor. She seemed to be acting strange, as though she didn't want to look at me or comfort me like the others did. She sat down on the side of the bed and looked at me as if she had bad news. She said, "David, we've found a lesion on your brain. It's a five by six by seven-centimeter lesion, and it looks as though it could be cancerous. It appears that it is most likely malignant, but we'll need to do some further testing to discover that. I just wanted you to know that this is what we're looking at right now." Then, as quickly as she came, she left. I never saw her again.

Corey slowly moved over to me and sat on the bed. He put his hand on top of mine. I sat there in silence, but this silence seemed so incredibly loud. Every thought I had about a person, place, phone call, project, was interrupted with the *BOOM* of the black, smudgy, oily, permanent stamp of brain cancer. How do I explain this to Amy? *(BOOM)* BRAIN CANCER. What about my mom? *(BOOM)* BRAIN CANCER. What about Dot&Cross? *(BOOM)* BRAIN CANCER. What about— *(BOOM)* BRAIN CANCER. Tears started to fall. No more words. No more thoughts. Corey silently got up and whispered he'd leave me to myself for a few minutes. He exited the room, and I started to weep. Loudly.

I had no idea. I had no clue this thing was living and breathing inside of me. I thought about having to tell my wife and my loving, crying mother. I thought about telling my family, my friends, and even my future kids. But what if this tumor takes me? What if I die early? I thought about what I would and would not accomplish with my life. I thought about how my parents and sisters would handle this news. I thought about how my friends and my company would handle this news. But all those thoughts fell flat when I realized that *one day I won't think anymore.*

I wanted to run but knew I wasn't fast enough. I wanted to hide but knew there was no place hidden enough. I wanted to scream but knew it wouldn't be loud enough. I wanted this moment to be a dream, but it was reality. I couldn't handle this news; it was too much. Everything was too much. Snot was running into my mouth and juicy tears were streaming down my face as my seemingly cancer ridden arms lay helplessly at my side. Maybe I should get up and walk, but my cancer ridden legs couldn't carry me. I felt broken. I felt lied to. I felt unbelievably furious.

I wanted to say something but couldn't, and not because of this tumor, but because I had nothing to say. And like a burning plane amid dark billows of smoke, I went screeching downward, deteriorating into nothingness as I hit the ground. There was only one person who deserved to hear my silent screams: "God, you son of a bitch. You, who created me and knew full goddamn well—even as I was curled peacefully in my mother's womb—that I'd develop cancer one day, who knows how many days I have left, who is aware of the innermost feelings of my heart. How's this for the innermost feeling of my heart? GOD, YOU ARE A FUCKING JOKE! FUCK YOU!"

But then, two minutes later, that thought passed, just as every thought does. And that was the last moment I questioned the existence of God, because, for whatever reason, I knew better.

The first call I made was to Amy. I said hello. I heard her repetitive worrying questions about me as my breath shortened knowing what I was about to say. I hated to report this news to anyone, let alone her.

"I have...I have a brain tumor. I have cancer."

I can't remember what she said after that. But I do remember her saying she'd immediately cancel her photography workshop she was holding the following day and take the next flight to San Francisco. I tried to argue, explaining she didn't need to cancel it and that she could catch up with me afterwards, but she wouldn't hear of it. She was on her way.

My parents, who were visiting my sister and her husband in Slovakia, went into action. My father, a physician's assistant, went online, searching for numbers, seeking potential answers, making calls, and ordering whomever was on the other end of the phone to explain what the next step would be. My mother started packing their clothes. My sister started planning her departure from Bratislava, as Michael, my brother-in-law, began researching the best neurosurgical hospitals in the country.

I wrote my first cancer blog post at Jump David Jump. In that post, I tried to explain that my life was in God's hands. Brett was still with me, so he looked it over, making edits to make it somewhat readable, and then told me it was my job to hit the "publish" button.

Now the world knew.

The next day I met with a doctor who informed me they wanted to do surgery immediately. But my dad had received word of this from afar and requested a pause to ask for a second opinion from Mayo Clinic Hospital. Kent, our family's friend from Omaha who is a pediatrician, agreed, and we immediately made plans to leave Stanford for Mayo Hospital in Rochester, Minnesota.

Amy, Brett, and I flew out to Rochester where I would have a second opinion on what to do next. Donald Miller emailed me and told me about a local guy, Andy Cass, who would be able to pick us up at the airport and take us to a home owned by members of his church. And sure enough, when we landed, Andy took us to the peaceful and quiet home of Steven and Jeanne Wilson. It was such an amazing place, located in the quiet backwoods of Minnesota. When we walked into their home, they offered to feed us and told us they would provide whatever we needed during our stay there.

We sat down in our room and started unpacking. I got out my computer to check up on all of my well-wishes and noticed I had received an email from Christophe Julliard, Vice President of Quality and Planning at Sofitel Hotels, who was concerned about why I didn't fill out their guest survey. His email said:

Dear David,

Recently, we sent you an invitation to complete a Guest Satisfaction Survey concerning your stay with us at Sofitel San Francisco Bay, where you checked out on June 07, 2009. We noticed that you did not have time to complete the survey. We are concerned that you may not have responded because we have somehow failed to live up to your expectations. At Sofitel, we are committed to providing a superior guest experience to each and every one of our customers. Please take a few minutes to tell us how well we met your expectations. Thank you again for choosing Sofitel, and I look forward to hearing about your stay with us.

Sincerely,

Christophe Julliard, Vice President Quality and Planning, Sofitel Business and Leisure Hotels North America

I simply had to respond.

Dear Christophe,

I apologize for not completing my Guest Satisfaction Survey upon my check-out on June 7, 2009. However, you are indeed correct that I did not respond, considering I lacked ample time to complete the survey. Around checkout time on the 7th, I hurriedly exited the hotel in an ambulance. Please do not be concerned that you have somehow failed to live up to my expectations. In fact, the opposite is true! You have exceeded them! While I was staying at your hotel, your Cancer Detection System worked like a charm. After years of being completely unaware, your hotel helped me discover a pesky tumor that had been growing in my brain for years. Had I not stayed at your hotel, it is completely possible I never would have made use of your detection tool! (To clarify, by tool I mean the concrete slab in your hotel bar that I smacked my head on). Expectations = Exceeded! In addition, I truly enjoyed your in-house olive bread and pesto sauce. And that means quite a bit because typically I am not a fan of pesto.

However, I do feel obligated to tell you that in the moments after my grand mal seizure, while being wheeled through your lobby on a stretcher (once again, the hurry I mentioned), I did notice there were some leaves that had blown into the pool. As VP of Quality and Planning, I imagine this would fall below your standards. I assume when I return to your hotel next time, this matter will be taken care of.

Regards,

David Wenzel, Hotel Guest, Room 607, June 1–7, 2009

FIVE
BANANA CHICKEN BIOPSY

"MORE LIKE A HEAD-ON CAR CRASH," I said.

Of course, I had never known what that actually felt like, but when asked, I told them the seizure my body experienced created extremely intense pain across my entire body. That initial seizure caused my opposing muscles, like my biceps and triceps for example, to constantly pull against each other, placing stress on my humerus bone during that five-minute seizure. It's not uncommon for people to even snap their bones in half as their opposing muscles flex against each other. This had happened across my entire body, and I felt as though I had just survived an overwhelming head-on car crash. But the doctors had given me intense pain pills, which I loved swallowing every four hours.

My parents arrived in Minnesota and had researched a place for us to stay for the upcoming days ahead. The Nazarene Well House was a Christ-centered place for patients of Mayo who are staying in Rochester. It is funded yearly by those with connections to Mayo who know the care is among the best in the world, so they provide a place for visitors to stay at a minimal rate. Our entire group eventually ended up at the Nazarene Well House: Amy, Mom and Dad; my younger sister, Heather, and her husband, Michael; my sister, Angie, and her two girls, Lily and

Anabelle; and Amy's oldest sister, Angela Hunsberger (also a nurse), who came out to provide support and encouragement.

My social media was blowing up. Everyone was sending me emails or commenting on my pages. Don Miller even offered to write all of my thank you letters for me. We met many of the individuals staying at the Well House, including a lovely elderly woman, Donna, whose granddaughter had recently died. We met another couple, whose youngest daughter was fighting her own battle with cancer. And I remember the day when they came back to the Well House in tears. They had lost their little girl.

Amy and I, in some attempt to handle this news, would go on long riverside walks together. The conversation ranged from our future kids, to family, to doctors, and to the conventional treatments I would receive. Then we would go to sleep in our small hotel-esque bedroom with a miserably uncomfortable bed. Late one night, one of the other patients who was attending Mayo to deal with her mental issues, opened our door and snuck in. She scared Amy and I half to death at first, but then she showed us a small stuffed bear and told us it made her feel better and now she wanted to give it to me.

The next day we went to Mayo Clinic Hospital, where we met with Dr. Frederick Meyer, the head of its brain department, as well as the chairperson of Mayo Clinic, which had the number-one ranked neuroscience department in the country. He told us the same news we had previously heard at Stanford, but he wanted to do his own MRI scans, as well as perform a full analysis of my health before moving forward. Dr. Meyer offered his concerns. He told us the mass was sitting between the two areas of the left temporal lobe associated with verbal speech and the processing of language. These communicating neural fibers (telephone wires, essentially) serve to connect these two areas. It is their responsibility to allow my brain to process and convert thoughts into an organized sentence that makes verbal sense when spoken (in other words, my ability to put the right words in the right order and speak them correctly as they to relate to the subject my brain is currently thinking about).

Dr. Meyer told us I had an oligodendroglioma that measured seven by six by five centimeters, a tumor that represented about 4 percent of all brain tumors. In his scientific opinion (and in my very loose words): My tumor had been there a while, maybe even ten years, and there seemed to be a malignancy, a "hot-spot," that was growing but buried beneath years of calcified, bone-hard tissue. In order to get to this area and remove it, he would need to work around and possibly remove some of this calcification. It would need to be an "awake surgery" during which I would be continually answering questions to actively measure the amount of brain being lost during the surgery. The difficult part was that this calcified mass was fused with, and surrounded, the two verbal areas of my brain and the delicate wires that connect them. These areas control the majority of comprehension and speech production. Surgery would be high risk, carrying a 20 percent chance of permanent speech deficit, so it should only be considered as a last option. If he felt he could remove 70 to 80 percent of this tumor, it would be worth the risk. However, he felt he could only remove about 40 percent of it. An attempt to remove any more could lead to permanent comprehension and speech production deficit. He could only see this as a final-straw option. He finalized his words by breathing deeply and saying this tumor is like "a chicken wire in the middle of your birthday cake, and any attempt to get the chicken wire out would destroy the cake."

When we opted out of this surgery, Dr. Meyer was relieved. He told us he didn't think it was a good idea either. To him, this tumor was inoperable. But before we could do anything else, he would need to perform a stereotactic biopsy, meaning they would drill a hole into my head and retrieve a sample of the tumor "hot-spot."

The night before I was to enter surgery, my sister Angie sent me an article by John Piper, called "Don't Waste Your Cancer," written on the eve of John's prostate surgery. John's first point was as follows:

> *This tumor was specifically designed for me by God…You will waste your cancer if you do not believe it is designed for you by God. It will not do to say that God only uses our cancer, but does not design it. What God permits, he permits for a reason. And that reason is his design. If God foresees molecular developments becoming cancer, he can stop it or not. If he does not, he has a purpose. Since he is infinitely wise, it is right to call this purpose a "design." If you don't believe your cancer is designed for you by God, you will waste it.*

I wasn't necessarily *for* this concept of God, but I also wasn't completely *opposed* to it. It was simply a statement, made by a great man of faith, who was dealing with his own battle of cancer. But his statement also meant that God had permitted this cancer for me. What does that even mean? I had no idea what God was going to accomplish by giving me, a twenty-seven- year-old unknown kid from the Midwest, an inoperable brain tumor.

The next day I woke up for my biopsy. I had noticed that patients who spent time at the hospital were always wandering around in their pajamas, but I determined that would not be me. So, when I arrived at five in the morning with Amy and my dad, I was properly dressed for the day. Belt on, hair done, cologne sprayed—everything. We were in a small waiting room, and eventually they came in to get me, first asking, "Name and birthday?" I went into the first room where they asked me to change into my surgical gown. Then a new nurse—also asking, "Name and birthday?"—took some blood and inserted two separate needles that would be used for IVs. I still have a scar from the wide-gauge needle they used.

They had me lie down flat on a patient bed for ten to twenty minutes before someone came back and picked me up. "Name and birthday?" They wheeled me into the pre-op room and parked me in the middle of a room filled with patients all prepared for surgery that morning. My anesthesiologist came over to me ("Name and birthday?") and gave me my first dose of the "light" stuff. Then he asked me which side of my head the tumor was in. I was shocked to hear he didn't know but told him it was the left side. He said, "Point at it." So, I raised my left hand and pointed at the left side of my head. Then he lightly grabbed my hand, pulled out a blue sharpie, and made an "X" on my left forearm. Then he turned and walked away, leaving me confused.

I looked around to see if anyone else had blue sharpie markings on them. It was so strange for me to see at least ten other patients, dressed in white, lying on their backs with no nurses around. For about twenty minutes we lay there, all in complete silence. I felt as if we knew each other on some bizarre level, each of us scared, lying next to each other in quiet support.

A pre-op nurse entered the room and approached a patient. "Name and birthday?" Then they wheeled him off. After a few more minutes, I heard it again, "Name and birthday?" Again, "Name and birthday?" Before I knew it, I was the last patient in the room. I was starting to feel as though I'd been forgotten about, when the nurse finally entered the room and came up to me.

"Name and birthday?"

"David Wenzel, October 15th, 1981."

She paused. I looked up at her as she eyed my chart, then looked back at my face. She said, "This might sound random, but were you just featured on Jasmine Star's blog?" Silence. "Umm. Yes?" Apparently, this medical student, in the deepest halls of Mayo's surgical center, was assigned to my case and recognized me as I lay there in my bed, covered in white gowns with a surgical head piece covering my hair. She was also a photographer and had read my story two days earlier on

Jasmine's blog. And now there she was, comforting me before my surgery.

I felt my heart fill up again, knowing I wasn't alone and that somehow word spreads in the most interesting and oftentimes backwards ways. She wheeled me toward my surgical room and comforted me as we made small talk. I was so shocked by all of this that I could only imagine her as my guardian angel, sent by God in my moment of need.

She wheeled me into a white room with about four or five people, each tending to their own responsibilities. As they were positioning me, one of the surgical assistants turned around and, in shock, said, "Oh! We're doing this one?" Not exactly the thing you want to hear from the team who is about to use power tools to cut your skull open and stick long sharp things into your brain. Then, while explaining to me what they were about to do, they pointed at the images on the TV screens above me to show how they had digitally recreated my brain. They constructed a 3-D map by piecing together the results of my functional MRIs and x-rays to avoid the active portions of my brain involved in spelling, language, cognition, and memory. They placed me in my final position, locking my head down in this heavy metal contraption so that I would be unable to move. Again, they explained they were about to drill a pencil-sized hole in my head and place a needle into the hot-spot of my tumor and draw out four different samples for examination.

My anesthesiologist explained they were about to insert the "heavy" dose into my IV. As they injected it, my nurse spoke, "Okay David, you're going to go to sleep now. Where do you want to go in your dream?"

A question? Seriously? Geez, I don't know. I said the first thing I could think of: "Tokyo."

"Okay," she said, as she placed the mask over my face.

I felt the numbness starting to settle in as I thought more about my answer. I imagined the loud noises, the honking horns, the pollution, the signs in different languages. What a horrible place to dream of! I mumbled, "No, no, no…" Alarmed, they quickly took my mask off, concerned something was going wrong: "David? Are you okay?" Deep into the heavy stuff, about to pass out, I said, "No…Not Tokyo. I…I want…I want New Zealand." Realizing this wasn't a medical issue, they breathed a massive sigh of relief and simply put the mask back over my face.

I didn't dream shit.

The resection of the tumor was a success. As the anesthesiologists were bringing me out of my deep sleep, I felt like I weighed a million pounds sitting on a lumpy sofa watching random thoughts parade through my mind. I couldn't put my finger on any of them though. I started trying to mumble something. The nurses saw this and told me, "David, you did great! Wonderful job!" Then in my garbled, post-brain-surgery voice, I said, "Knock, knock."

Every single person in the entire room paused and looked at me in shock. The nurse hesitantly responded, "Who's there?"

ME: *Banana.*

NURSE: *Banana who?*

ME: *Banana Chicken.*

The room looked back at the nurse to hear her response, which never came. Then I asked if she understood the joke my niece Lily had told me a few days before. She said no. I told her I didn't either.

They took me back to the ICU, where I would be monitored through the night. I arrived in a very nice room meant for two people, but it was just me. About an hour into my stay, I asked my nurse if I could get up to use the bathroom. She looked at me and politely laughed as she informed me I'd had a catheter inserted and could just pee right there. I'm sure my response gave away the fact I had no idea they placed a catheter in me after I was passed out in the surgical room. She walked away chuckling as my hand slowly reached down and inspected the aftermath. *Ah crap*, I thought. *I bet my guardian angel from heaven handled my unconscious junk to put this contraption in me.*

Amy spent the night with me, and I'm so glad she did because it turned out to be the most frustrating night ever. I was lassoed to the bed with monitors of all sorts alerting the nurses in case my heart stopped or slowed down. At the beginning of the night, the alarm would go off if my heart dropped below sixty beats a minute. It beeped. And it beeped loudly, so someone would hear it and come running. The nurse came back to adjust the alarm to go off at fifty beats a minute. Again, my heart rate dropped below fifty beats a minute. BEEP! Then forty-five. BEEP! Then forty. BEEP! I was told the machine couldn't go any lower than forty beats a minute. So, the night after my open-brain surgery, I was unable to sleep because of the medical equipment hooked up to me. I became so frustrated that at four in the morning, when my alarm started beeping again, I start screaming, "GET IN

HERE, I'M REDLINING! I MIGHT BE DEAD BY NOW!"

A few days later I went to see Dr. Uhm, my radiologist who had analyzed my brain sample. He told me I had Grade II Oligodendroglioma with a co-deletion of the 1p/19q chromosomes. The co-deletion of these chromosomes meant that my body would be much more receptive to the chemotherapy that he would soon prescribe for me. I knew I liked Dr. Uhm when he began explaining my situation like this:

"There are three of you sitting in this room with me. Let's pretend there is an assassin attempting to kill one of you. What is the best way he could possibly do it? Well, theoretically, he could..."

I was sold. I didn't even care what else he had to say. But he explained all of the potential outcomes of my biopsy and detailed what the best and worst scenarios could be. Thirty minutes later, I was well informed about the nature of the cancer in my head, but somehow, he managed to explain it all to me through an array of analogies including parking garages, a single magical car with hundreds of accelerators and brake pedals, his daughter's grades, Olympic marathons, and his wife's feelings regarding the final installation of the wood flooring in his new house.

There were so many different medical tests and documents to sign, but I was so pleased I didn't have to deal with them. The only thing I had to do was sign the occasional paper after receiving a head nod from someone I shared DNA with. Above all things on this earth, I hate paperwork. My mom and dad were dealing with my insurance company to understand the extravagant costs that were piling up. Later they came to inform me that my insurance company had turned down my claim. Strangely enough, the insurance company couldn't find any of my past medical documents to prove there were no "previous symptoms." I had been so healthy my entire life that the only documented medical problem I had ever had was a childhood ear infection, which only required a quick visit to the ER.

We all sat and thought. Where on earth can we find my name on any type of medical record? Then it hit me! In elementary school they kept records! My father contacted Hickory Hill Elementary School in Papillion and heroically located my past medical documents. And by documents, I mean he found one and a half pages of handwritten notes passed along by my grade-school nurse, Mrs. Kathy Roehrig, who detailed my medical history from 1987–1997. First, we couldn't believe they actually held onto these handwritten "official records," and second, we realized several ridiculous, intricate details of my elementary school experience. A few notable entries included:

Oct 24, 1988 — Scraped hand on playground. Put water on it. Ice pack. Sent back to class.

Sep 25, 1990 — Sunburn on right shoulder. Ice pack. Sent back to class.

Sep 25, 1990 (Same day) — Complaint of another student slapping sunburn on right shoulder. Ice pack. Sent back to class.

Immediately, it all came back to me! Ann Romjue had slapped my shoulder after I told her I was sunburned! But that slap brought on another opportunity to leave class, so I told the teacher I had to return to receive more "treatments." It appears Hickory Hill Elementary School's nursing system was indeed quite simple but, apparently, well documented. But after the insurance company received a copy of these hand-written notes including my headaches (also most likely fake) captured by our nurse, they agreed to cover all the overwhelming and still increasing medical costs, which made everyone breathe a sigh of relief. This ridiculous, yet historically accurate, piece of paper brought back memories of my trips to the nurse's office. It didn't matter if you had a broken leg, a raspy throat, or an arm cut off, you came back to class with a frozen dish-sponge in a Ziploc bag with a brown paper towel around it. I can still smell the mold.

Amy and I privately discussed what we individually believed regarding miraculous healing and what we were taught growing up in the Baptist church, as well as what we learned in recent years. She was in complete support of God's full healing. I explained I didn't refuse to believe in miracles, but I'd also never seen anyone healed in person. I always "heard" these stories but never "saw" them. But after learning of my own cancer, I became a quick believer. Knowing this tumor was inoperable and hearing I only had five to seven years left to live, I had to believe there was another way.

We gathered my family to sit in a circle on the floor of the Nazarene Well House basement. Amy and I talked through our previous and current feelings for believing in miraculous healing. We went around the circle and asked every individual if they were willing to believe with us in this. When it came to my mother, she started crying and admitted that when her mother, Granny Louise Tate, died of ovarian cancer two decades before, she had never honestly held out hope for complete miraculous healing. The odds of healing were too overwhelming to hold out hope for. Her mother's illness seemed too big for her to wrap her arms around. Louise was nearly seventy and lived a full life, but now Mom couldn't believe this was happening to me, her own son. My parents had each gone through spiritual awakenings in the past twenty years and agreed to stand with us in belief that God can and would work a miracle in my life. We all agreed, sitting in a circle, that yes, I was diagnosed with Grade II Oligodendroglioma, an inoperable brain tumor, but all of us equally agreed together that God, in his mercy, would give me a full life. We all agreed we would leave that circle, as well as the state of Minnesota, on the same page.

The flights were long, and my head was in serious pain due to the changes in altitude and its effect on my swollen brain. I landed in my familiar Grand Rapids Airport a full month after I left for San Francisco. Amy and I exited the terminal to find a group of my dearest friends waiting for me with balloons. It was a welcome-home celebration with Sonny, Corey, Brett, Kelly, Ben, Chuck, and Holly. I never expected to get a warm welcome like this, but it was only the beginning of the love I would feel upon returning home.

It made me think of all the love I was surrounded by through this entire experience. When trouble found me, my business partner, Brett, was at my side and even prolonged his trip to stay with me. I was helped by my wife who canceled a twenty-person photography conference to fly to San Francisco immediately. My parents had skipped a planned trip to Paris to rush to Minnesota, and some dear family friends, the Amstutzes, had given up their holiday to stand next to my hospital bed. I was surrounded by my own family flying in from around the world, dear friends waiting in airports to greet me. Lasagnas were delivered in the trunks of cars, beautiful flowers left on our doorstep, and random envelopes filled with money and labeled "Groceries" appeared. And there were hugs from local store attendants down the street and also business partners, who, without a single complaint, picked up my workload.

It was a life-altering moment to see these people, some I didn't even know, who cared about me and the actions they took to show it. It made me think of how much I wanted to live my life differently. I wanted to be like Bob Goff and show my love the way he showed his. Everyone shrugged it off, shaking their head and saying their kindness shown was incredibly small, but I saw it as evidence of so much more. While living my perfect life, I had never comprehended the idea that, out of nowhere, any one of us could be hit by a bus, suffer a heart attack, or be diagnosed with a terminal and inoperable brain tumor. But right now, it was me who had to learn I may or may not have five to seven years left to live. My question now was, "What will I do with that time?"

SIX
WE'LL MEET AGAIN

"WE'LL MEET AGAIN" was the song I couldn't get out of my head. Immediately, I knew Johnny Cash's version will be the final song at my funeral. And maybe I'll have Bob Goff come and speak about my life. I can't imagine Amy would want to say anything, but I'm sure some of my friends will. Of course my dad will want to talk, and it will most likely include some type of YouTube montage video he was tweaking just before he gets up to speak. I definitely don't want a typical funeral. It should be just another little party my dead body throws for all my friends. People should have fun while they're there, eating pizza, drinking beer, and telling stories. I should look into putting my personal keepsakes in piñatas.

It was strange to be thinking about these things only a few weeks after learning I have a brain tumor. But now, when I lay in bed late at night, my mind was fixated on it. *If I have been given five to seven years left to live, why would I be considering who will DJ my funeral? Where would I be when I passed away? What would be the condition of my body? Would I be at home? In a hospital? On a flight? Hopefully, not driving.* I became fascinated with death. But not the being dead part; I was interested in the step-by-step process I would go through to become dead. Would I drop dead in the middle of a seizure one day? I'd heard of that happening before. Would I fade away, slowly forgetting how to talk, how to remember? Would I not recognize Amy when she walks into the room, mistaking her for a nurse? I'm not necessarily scared at this point, just extremely curious about how my body will slowly start to shut down.

I'm still shocked at how I went from living my life to considering my death through one single incident. But this type of news changes everything. It changed what's important to me. It rearranged how I think about God, life, and death. I thought about my parents: *Will they watch me die?* I've heard that's the worst thing for a parent to go through. I thought about Amy as a widow. Will she stand next to me as I fade away, supporting me like a rock as she had done when she canceled her conference and flew to San Francisco?

If I hadn't declared my condition on my blog, I imagine the general public would have never known. I've always been the type of person to be concerned with how people perceive me, so no matter what I was doing, I put on a good show. But this wasn't a show. By being open and curious about my future, I hoped to provide a clear look into my battle with cancer. I would be so appreciative if I were able to read about it from another person—an honest story about the process, the changes in the body, what chemotherapy and radiation feel like, and how it affects the human body.

When I thought about what it would take for me to be that person, it gave me hope. I was no longer sad about my life being put on the line because now it would serve a purpose. I knew Amy had enough money to take care of herself. Not to mention the publicity of my death would be great for her business. And of course, our families would be there to support her through it.

But I'd never really thought of the process of dying before. I'm not scared of dying. I am convinced Jesus has saved my soul and I will spend eternity with him, next to my beloved granddaddy and grandmother. And in the end, I know the rest of my family will join me there. Overall, it seems the afterlife process is pretty much taken care of.

Still, I can't deny the fact that I now have a unique story to tell. I'm now the strategic filmmaker/writer who only has a few years of his life left. What will he do? How will he spend his time? Does he throw it all away and move to a foreign land? Does he become a monk and live in harmony with God and nature? Does he keep pressing away at his job pretending nothing ever happened? Does he switch jobs to pursue the one he always wanted? I must admit I considered all of these options.

But again and again, my mind returned to the question of "Why?" Why do I have cancer? Did I bring this upon myself with my lifestyle? Why should I have to die when I have been trying to live a full life, Tits and Ass style? Why am I being told I only have a few years left when I had always been so healthy? Never had a cavity, never broken a bone, and never needed to visit a doctor. And it still seemed I had incredible brain function.

However, looking back over the past year, I realized that the noises surrounding me in the office had bothered me. Sirens, knocks on doors, any type of inconsistent sound threw me off my game. I even had to change the music I listened to while working. I moved from music with words to classical music with no words. The lyrics were messing up my thought processes. At that time, I probably thought my musical palette was advancing. Guess not.

The real core of my questioning landed on God. So, I asked Him, "God, did you allow this?" "Did you create this tumor specifically for me?" "Did you simply stand by as you did with Job when you set the Devil loose on him?" Job whose crop was burnt, whose possessions were stolen by bandits, whose body was ravaged by diseases, whose children were killed. I wanted to ask God, as Job had also asked, "Did I do something wrong? Did you make some kind of pact with the Devil so that he could have his way with me?"

I wanted to yell at God using Job's actual words, *"Is not calamity for the unrighteous, and disaster for the workers of iniquity? Does not he see my ways and number all my steps? If I have walked with falsehood and my foot has hastened to deceit, if my step has turned aside from the way and my heart has gone after my eyes, and if any spot has stuck to my hands, then let me sow and another eat, and let what grows for me be rooted out."*

But in the end, God puts Job in his place. I could almost hear God thundering these words at me with His stern voice, *"Dress for action like a man; I will question you, and you will make it known to me."* And, like Job, I imagined cowering from the power of God, quietly responding, *"Behold, I am of small account; what shall I answer you? I lay my hand on my mouth."*

I know God feels my pain. I believe Him to be a loving God and, as with many people who have walked this cancer road ahead of me, He has heard every prayer, every promise, and every bargain put on the table before Him. But the simple knowledge of that fact nearly made me not care about praying anymore. When I sat in my bed and earnestly prayed that God would miraculously remove my tumor, I simply thought, *God knows I have cancer. If He allowed it, then He knows what he is going to do with it next. And if He knows that, then there's nothing I can do to change it. So, why pray?*

Yet while I believe in a God who knows everything before it happens, I also believe that my participation is required. And if that's the case, I must take action. And when I looked to the Bible, I saw examples of individuals who convinced God to "change His mind." Can we really do that? Can we actually interact with God to change His mind? If so, did He know we were going to do that and initially sandbag us with His fake plan? After my four years at a Christian university, all I learned was enough to make me ask dangerous questions in times like this. But like Abraham, one of those who convinced God to change his mind, I can firmly say that God, through all of this, has never left me. Of course, He's never shown me what's coming next, but I know he hasn't turned his back on me. He's just slowly introducing me to the next chapter of my life.

I can't deny the fact I constantly felt undergirded by Him. I knew that in the middle of all of this, He was right there next to me. I can't explain it, but I felt He was looking directly at me, quietly watching my every move. I wanted to complain, "God! What have you done?" But like any knowing and loving father, He would look at me with peace in His eyes and continually reply, "Wait, David. Your story is just starting to get good."

My doctors at Mayo had connected me with their partners at the University of Michigan Comprehensive Cancer Center and assigned me a doctor in Ann Arbor to consult with. Amy and I drove the two hours from Grand Rapids to the cancer center, where I was asked for yet another MRI. After this, all of my Michigan doctors compared notes and told me they wanted to create my radiation plan to be dispensed at a location in Grand Rapids, where I would have to go every day for six weeks.

Eventually, I was passed over to a young physician whom I would continue to see on each of my returns. Each visit, she took more MRIs showing the tumor just hanging out. Not growing. Not shrinking. Just slowly, painlessly, killing my brain. We talked again about why surgery wasn't an option and about different types of radiation and chemotherapy. But one day, my new physician told me something I was unprepared to hear. She once had cancer (though not of the brain) and had gone through a very similar conventional strategy we were discussing for myself. It was most likely a vulnerability move she uses to draw cancer patients closer to her—her ace card for unruly patients like me. I'm sure many patients have previously said, "Oh, you've had cancer as well? Then, of course, I'll do whatever you want me to do." Not me.

Part of me hated this idea of conventional therapy. That meant I was just another patient, waiting in the same line, following the same plan, and receiving the same pills to combat the same conditions. Deep down I felt something better must exist. I wanted to be well prepared for what was coming my way, so I started asking around. How can I survive this treatment and potentially thrive through radiation and chemo? I received some great answers including an intense amount of Vitamin C through an IV, specific nutrient pills, and seriously restricted vegan or raw diets. I learned that if I was going to fight this cancer on my own, it was not going to be easy or cheap.

God never seems to call us to do simple things—only things that require us to follow Him—knowing full well we don't have the answers to survive on our own. But those are the stories the Bible is full of. Those are the stories that God loves to tell. I was very vocal about my faith through my blog, causing readers to send me emails asking me how I can believe in a God that would allow me this type of agony and pain. But suddenly that question didn't make sense to me. If we didn't have pain, we would essentially be living in some type of heaven here on earth. And I know this isn't Heaven. That true heavenly existence, which I could now sense in front of me and that I could hear quietly calling me, is the reason I want to make different decisions here on Earth. It's why I want to love. It's why I want to make the best with what I have. It's why I want to start thinking more about those who don't have enough to eat or drink. Because one day we're all going to show up in Heaven and, as Jesus said, the things we did for the least of these, were the things we did for him. This nearly unbelievable news of my cancer wasn't just another reminder that we are not in Heaven yet, but a great reminder of the person I wanted to become here on Earth.

On Amy's and my next trip to the hospital, a nurse explained the high likelihood that my chemotherapy treatment would make me sterile. The nurse then pulled out a small cup and informed me that I would ejaculate into it. Then they would freeze my sperm for our use in the future. Amy and I looked at each other and nervously started laughing at this concept, not because it was funny, but because it was so overwhelmingly sad we had to have some other type of shared response. What does that procedure even look like? Would Amy come with me or would I do it by myself? Would I one day tell my future children they were conceived from my sensual trip to exam room four?

After that, I visited the radiation center. They explained how the procedure would go and discussed my radiation mask. The mask was a plastic head cover that could be locked down to keep my head still while they injected me with laser beams. They took a long slab of rigid plastic mesh and placed it over my face before they started applying hot wet rags to soften up the material. I'll never forget that feeling of my face being permanently pressed into this plastic mask. They held that mask up in front of my face, smiling, and somehow joyfully explained it would offer me a safer procedure. But I couldn't help but stare at it. It kinda looked like my head, but completely empty. It was just my facial features, my nose, my chin, and my forehead.

I thought I would be completely focused on God throughout this process, but I wasn't. I had somehow returned to a strange form of hopelessness in the months following this diagnosis. I felt that my path to dealing with this cancer was a dud, and going through this procedure made me feel just as hollow as that mask looked.

It made me think of my previous trips to Mayo Hospital or the Michigan cancer center. I always began in the cancer therapy waiting room, looking at the people, each experiencing this new world of conventional treatment, as though I were an astronaut landing on a foreign planet. I was surrounded by people in wheelchairs missing limbs, elderly people with patches over their skin, former businessmen now bald and weak, and cancer-laden mothers whose kids were running amuck. This room, covered in miserable art, week-old newspapers, and pots of life-ending coffee, struck me as such a place of misery, of lost hope, and of pain. *Is this my future?*

Part of me felt that I would be exactly like them one day. But I won't be an elderly person or a small child. I'll be that middle-aged guy in the corner, the one who you could tell was, in his day, somewhat attractive. But now his sunken eyes and half-head of hair has turned him into a shadow. He's grown a shitty beard because he no longer takes care of himself. His mismatched socks match his mismatched sentences, if he ventures to say anything at all. After being sick for so long, he's vomited himself gaunt, so his clothes are now far too big for him. He's brought his own slippers because he's all-too familiar with the local footwear. He's simply following his doctor's orders to keep him alive when, in the end, he can't help but think the best way for him to go is to have a seizure in his bed and never wake up.

This thought of my slow degradation was always lurking a half-step behind me. Fear was setting in, a fear not of death but the act of dying. I have been told by every doctor I've seen that this tumor will kill me. It is only a matter of how and when. I have been given a deadline of five to seven years. Too much time for Amy and I to spend our money eating, drinking, and traveling the world, yet enough time to be required to go back to work and act like nothing ever happened. I was stuck in the middle, requiring my best efforts to keep on living and working, while simultaneously joining the weakened masses in the cancer treatment waiting lobby, being radiated, throwing up from chemotherapy, jerking off into clear sanitary cups, slowly dying, knowing that any day could be my last.

Dear God, I wondered, *what happens next? I'm not fully alive. I'm not fully dead. I have simply arrived in my purgatory.* And soon my medical saviors, chemotherapy and radiation, would strip away the elements of myself that I felt made me who I am, or who I thought I was. *I don't want to go out like that.* Some days I spent in hope, trusting that God had not yet forgotten me and repeating His words of healing, while on other days, I wished I could skip all this rigmarole and get to the end. To start my eternity now by strolling through the gates of Heaven and offering God the finger, as I hear those words from Johnny Cash being sung at my funeral:

> *"We'll meet again, don't know where. Don't know when. But I know we'll meet again some sunny day. Keep smiling through, just like you always do, till the blue skies drive the dark clouds far away. And will you please say hello to the folks that I know. Tell 'em I won't be long. And they'll be happy to know that as you saw me go, I was singing this song. We'll meet again, don't know where, don't know when, but I know we'll meet again some sunny day."*

And maybe in that last chorus, you could all stand up, hold hands, and sing it together.

SEVEN
THE EYES NEVER LIE

THE OLD BUILDING LOOKED LOPSIDED FROM THE SIDEWALK. But after double-checking the address on Eastern Avenue, I wandered up the musty stairwell. I smelled something—not patchouli, but something exotic enough to remind me how far I'd traveled from the sterile halls of Mayo Clinic Hospital. At the top of the stairs I found a typical client waiting room filled with old magazines, fake plants, and a tiny water fountain recycling dirty white noise. The purpose of my visit was to discover a proper diet to help me through my chemotherapy and radiation treatments.

Micah, a naturopath suggested by a friend, entered from the back hallway looking like he had just rolled out of bed. Later, I realized this was his everyday look. He kindly greeted me, shook my hand, and invited me back to his office. As I walked behind him, I peeked into all the rooms with open doors. In one I heard recordings of chanting monks softly playing. In another I saw a massage bed in front of a table with unlit candles, carefully arranged oils, and what appeared to be tuning forks lying in perfect rows. I'd unknowingly walked into a hippie torture chamber. I sighed and wondered, *Why am I here?*

My daily existence orbited around that lingering unanswered question, *why?* As a patient, you can ask your doctors absolutely anything, as long as it starts with what or when or where, but never why. For example, "Why do I have a tumor in my head?" Asking *why* leaves too much space for fuzzy answers, so doctors quietly shuffle those questions away, reminding you to be a good patient who follows instructions. They want your mind focused on their strategy and not on the stories people tell you of what worked for their grandmother. But when a person with an open mind stands up and honestly yells "Why is this happening?", I imagine the universe must stand at attention and intercede, possibly even offering a new compass heading directly to Eastern Avenue.

Micah closed the door behind us, a practice that typically makes me double-check for other exits. He smiled, approached me, and reached out his arms to wrap me in a hug. After a diagnosis like mine, one's body becomes public property, like a pregnant woman's. Many complete strangers have felt the need to place their hands on my head or grab my shoulders out of pity. But Micah's hug didn't feel inappropriate at all for a first-time meeting. It was warm and honest. I liked it. I would pay good money to learn to hug like him.

I sat down in Micah's office and quickly took in the room. I noticed shelves of bottles bearing names I couldn't pronounce, teas with images of wild flowers, and books about roots. This was the exact opposite of what I had previously experienced at Mayo and the University of Michigan Cancer Center. Micah wore no shoes, smelled of mystical oils, possessed a scruffy beard, and had what I assumed to be a self-installed nose ring. All he carried was an odd smile. His wide, close-mouthed grin seemed to wiggle through my chest and exit through my back, filling the room like helium inside a yellow balloon. The room was electrically charged with his presence, something I appreciated because my presence felt broken. I liked how I felt sitting in front of Micah.

I broke the silence by starting to talk—a nervous tick I inherited from my mother. I suggested we begin talking about radiation-friendly diets or any other tricks to survive the conventional treatment process. He told me we'd eventually get there, but he wanted to begin with his own methods. First, he explained that we would take close-up photos of my eyes and put together an integrated physical and emotional map of my life. I tried to hide my smirk. Apparently, these photos would display the mysteries of my body. This simple exchange made it perfectly clear to me why alternative medicine had received such a bad rap. Now I found myself on the complete opposite side of the medical world, in a lopsided building, hugging strangers, and snapping pictures of my baby-blues to determine my medical past. *Whatever. I can do this. Bring it on, Micah the Magician.*

We began with iridology, a practice of taking extreme close-up photos of your irises to catalog the physical and emotional history of your life. This sounded like solid joke fodder, and I began mentally selecting which friends I would recount this experience to over beers. After taking about forty photos, Micah uploaded them to his computer and briefly perused them. He eyed me across the table strangely and told me that I had some of the healthiest eyes he'd ever seen. Most people, Micah explained, have all sorts of deposits—tiny little discolored spots and fuzzy fibers extending from the pupil to the edge of the iris. He explained that stress, toxins, illness or even broken bones, especially early in life, create a permanent record in your eyes, like a mobile medical file.

Next, we checked out photos of my sclera (the white part around my iris), a similar practice called sclerology. This would be a better indicator of the current conditions in my body conducive to cancer growth. Much to my disbelief, Micah was actually able to show me small markings that indicate a propensity for "new growth" or a tendency toward cancer. He explained how the lines in my left eye created certain cancer patterns that pointed to a specific portion of my brain. Micah, who I imagine understands his patients' never-ending skepticism, swiveled a one-eighty in his chair to grab a book off the shelf. He opened it up and plopped it down in front of me. He turned his laptop around and showed me my photos. The strangely intrusive photos of my left eye, containing all the little red squiggly lines like an old trail map, followed a pattern. Of course there were regular lack of sleep or stress lines, but there were others, containing hooks or bends that, according to this book (most likely printed when I was in grade school), represented tissue prone to cancer activity in a specific portion of the left side of my brain.

I was in absolute shock. My mouth hung open as I analyzed the photos of my eyes versus the images in the book. I wanted to continue discussing them, but Micah had already moved on. There was something else in my sclera that bothered him. In fact, he said it was the most significant thing going on in my eye, even more noteworthy than the cancer markings. At the bottom interior corner of each of my eyes were intense lines extending toward my eyeball. He told me these lines were originating from my "emotional heart."

After my initial surprise at being shown accurate results from a procedure I previously would have laughed at, Micah invited me a bit further down the rabbit hole with the words "emotional heart." He flipped a few pages in the book to a page with that title. Knowing he'd stretched himself a bit past the unspoken first meeting boundary, he read the passage to himself before hesitantly asking, "Do you want to hear this?" I maintained my composure, paying special attention to not moving a single muscle in my face. I've always wanted to be the guy who could hear something and analyze it before choosing to accept or deny it. In my desire to appear like a fair-minded person, I nodded for him to continue.

Micah began, "While I don't know you at all, and this could be way off, these emotional heart markings point to a very specific thing. Typically, this means that a person isn't doing what they should be doing with their life. This incongruence creates stress between what your emotional heart wants versus what your reality actually looks like. It's indicative of people who have built a large wall around their heart, guarding their true selves against the fear of rejection. It typically means the truest heart doesn't engage with the world. These lines show up in people who feel they have some type of 'calling,' and oftentimes the lines are associated with lifelong feelings that the person must 'change the world' or 'make an impact.' But when this calling is ignored or repressed, an internal stress is created and these lines show up in the emotional heart because the person isn't meeting this deep need to fulfill their life's calling. Does any of this sound like you?"

My poker face gave way to an eye roll.

"Micah, of course I've been thinking about this. For the last six weeks, I've been reevaluating life with freakin' brain cancer; what it means for my marriage and determining the changes it may have on my career. I'm not at all surprised these lines are showing up so strongly. This cancer has thrown my whole life into question. And I don't think it's a huge deal that I've got a few emotional heart lines questioning my meaning in life because, honestly, I am."

So much for fair-mindedness.

As I undermined his "emotional lines" bit, it dawned on me that part of his craft was connecting with new clients. Similar to a psychic staring into a crystal ball, he needed to say something blandly true about everyone, like, "There are new opportunities on your horizon, and you need to take advantage of them!" or "You have experienced trauma. Pay me to help you!"

Micah calmly responded, "David, I understand your recent struggles have probably intensified these lines, but they aren't new. They are so strong it appears they've been developing for a very long time, likely since childhood. To be honest, these are some of the strongest emotional heart lines I've ever come across. If any of this resonates with you, then whatever you are dealing with seems to be a very old problem and you've been dealing with it for a very, very long time. If deep down you feel like you've been *set apart* from the rest of the world to accomplish a task, and this task is extremely important to your identity, then you must pursue it. I know you think I'm crazy, but I think it might even be strongly related to the presence and the growth of your tumor. In fact, this tumor might be your body getting your attention to redirect your purpose to do what you have known for quite some time you should be doing. Because up until now, it seems you've been ignoring it."

In the middle of that speech, he said those same two words that have been haunting me my entire life. But now they enraged me: "set apart." Immediately, I was filled with the kind of rage that surfaces when someone calls you out, forcing you to stand emotionally naked in front of them. I wanted to write him off and tell him his methodology was full of shit and that I would never be tricked into his psychic trap. I wanted to punch him in the mouth and storm out of the room. He didn't even know me and had absolutely no right to say any of those things to me.

But he was right. My eyes had sold me out. All of this anger served as my security guard who protected a deep wound. Micah saw right past the disguise that had fooled every other person in my life. I'd been fighting this battle with myself for as long as I could remember; now Micah was asking me if I was willing to stand up and deal with my childhood desire to be "set apart." If I did, I knew I'd be met with more failure, rejection, and heartache.

I couldn't do it. I couldn't agree to go there again.

This deep indignation from Micah triggered a familiar feeling that started swirling in my gut, the same overwhelming sensation that took over my body in the coffee shop as I listened to Arcade Fire's "My Body is A Cage." My stomach turned over. My chest clamped up. My throat tightened and began to suffocate me. My breathing sped up against my will, resulting in uncontrollable sobs as I tried to keep my body together.

"David, do you know what these emotional lines might represent?" Micah asked after watching me attempt to wrestle my emotions to the ground. I knew I could lie and he wouldn't call me out. But if I did, I would forever look back on this moment as another one when I chose to run. I reached up to wipe away my big, hot, angry tears, and I managed to calm my breathing and accepted my defeat.

I quietly replied, "Yes, I know what it is."

I dropped the mask I'd put on for the world. I began to explain the desires of my youth that no one but Amy knew. I told Micah that, for as long as I can remember,

I knew I was created to speak, to write, to be a communicator. When I was young, I thought I could become an actor—and *Election* seemed to echo that desire—but quickly I had realized I didn't want to "act" as someone else. I wanted to be me. So, as I got older, I noticed the thing that made me buzz with excitement, that kept me up at night and forced me out of bed in the morning, was sharing with groups of people. I loved every second I spent in front of large groups of people. Public speaking, one of most people's greatest fears, was my deepest joy. But I'd never been bold enough to pursue it further. I felt empty because I never had a unique personal story worth telling.

I sat thinking through these details in front of Micah with my brief life flashing before my eyes. I began to chuckle through my tears as I saw the underlying nature of my partnership with Dot&Cross. I had created a reality as close as possible to doing this very thing by communicating with others through developing content and writing scripts. Every single day I woke up and spoke through our clients. I was key in creating the blueprints of their projects, piggy-backing off their influence, and watching as others impacted the world around them. I was building environments where I helped other people do exactly what I desperately wanted to do. But I accomplished it all while never facing the risk of personal rejection that might result from displaying my own vulnerable heart. I had created my own perfect world, but I only haunted it as a ghost.

I explained this to Micah, burning through a box of tissues and getting more animated as my internal passions lined up. I began explaining the details of what my emotional heart was starving for, but Micah, quite rudely, interrupted me mid-sentence with a strange question.

"Wait. David, where is your tumor...exactly?" I thought we had already covered this, but maybe I never actually told him where it was. This specific detail had become incredibly important to him as he heard me explain my desires. I began repeating my diagnosis, the same story I'd learned to tell verbatim over the past six weeks.

"The tumor is a Grade II Oligoastrocytoma. It's seven by six by five centimeters and sits in the frontotemporal lobe of my left brain. Typically, doctors resect or remove tumors like this, but mine is shaped more like a tree branch. It looks like chicken wire that laces through important portions of my brain, so it's inoperable. A resection could cause severe harm to the speech and communication portions of my brain due to its location. The doctors essentially told me a failed resection would cause damage to the wires that connect these two areas, meaning I could lose the ability to comprehend new concepts and create speech. Oh, and the tumor is also kinda sitting on top of my right motor cortex, which controls the function of the right side of my body, which sucks because I'm right handed and I love to write and—"

I stopped talking. My eyes opened wider. For the first time, my confusing thoughts filed into order and clicked into place. I met Micah's gaze and saw his mouth hanging wide open. We both sat in silence as we considered the same outlandish thought. The starter pistol for my brain fired. My thoughts took off in a dead sprint. Could the stress I'd created by continually running from my own God-given purpose since childhood be the onset of this cancer? Could this internal friction have sparked the growth of the tumor in the one and only place I needed it most—my speech comprehension areas? Immediately, I reviewed my recent reasoning. Could God have *created* this? Could He, or even would He, *allow* this? Maybe John Piper was right. Maybe this cancer was specifically designed for me. Maybe God created this tumor to push me to confront my desire to make an impact on my world, to be "set apart."

Everything went into slow-mo. I closed my eyes as tight as possible. My logical brain was being asked to consider unscientific reasoning. I tried to control my mind, suspend all immediate judgments, hold back all medical explanations, and entirely accept this moment as it happened. I felt I should wrap my heart in thick orange safety rope before letting it sink into a giant unexplored sinkhole to discover whatever existed below my well-reasoned surface. I opened my eyes and looked at Micah, knowing exactly what he was thinking. But I wanted to hear the words from his mouth. I wanted him to speak the words born simultaneously in our respective guts. I braced for impact.

"Knowing full well that every doctor you've seen has said they have no idea what could have caused this tumor. Knowing that you have never received any dramatic trauma to the head as a child that could have caused this tumor. Is it possible that the stress your emotional heart has endured since you were a young child, from knowing exactly what you should be doing with your life—communicating truth—but never completely fulfilling this in your life, has somehow caused overwhelming friction within this exact portion of your brain? Is it possible that your deep and ongoing emotional struggle to fulfill your life's purpose may actually have opened the door for this cancer?"

"David," he continued. "I don't think radiation or chemotherapy will resolve this. And actually, I'm not entirely sure changing your diet or taking herbal supplements will work either. I'm not sure the root issue of this cancer is necessarily affecting your physical organs, as much as it is affecting your deeper sense of existence. If you want to be rid of this tumor, you must face this specific issue head on. The ongoing struggle to face this aspect of your life could be the main source of all your physical issues. David, your body has just hit the pause button. You can keep doing the things you've been doing or you can make this change, and—as strange as it may sound—potentially heal yourself."

Micah didn't seem like one to care about rules. I shouldn't have been surprised it only took him thirty minutes before he managed to ask the one forbidden question I was told never to ask, "Why is there a tumor in my brain?" If indeed there was a supernatural answer to this question of *why*, it would mean my cancer wasn't biologically blind or a "rare happenstance" as explained by doctors. This cancer had hunted me down and preyed on me as I unknowingly ran from it. This cancer was my own personal struggle keeping me from accomplishing exactly what I was put on this earth to do. If this was indeed the case, the previous moments of my life moments weren't happenstance at all; they were predetermined plot points leading me directly to Eastern Avenue.

My strong internal desires from an early age weren't bizarre at all. They were simply setting the stage for a story only now starting to open up. Dot&Cross wasn't just another job; it was preparation for my unknown future. My early morning encounter with Arcade Fire was a musical prophecy pointing directly toward this diagnosis. This was the reason I unexpectedly ended up in San Francisco at the Expert Academy. This was underlying the meaning of why I became so frustrated with the direction of my life that I had to escape to San Jose and spill Morrissey's prayerful song lyrics to Josh. There was a reason I took a one-hour train ride back to the hotel, arriving at 12:15 a.m., to meet the person who asked, "What type of expert are you?" And there was a comically distinct reason I responded with kung fu to perhaps the only person willing to fake a battle with me in the hotel lobby. Kung fu was why I whacked my head on a concrete pillar, unlocking the tumor that had been silently growing in my head for nearly ten years. Kung fu, the mockery of my actual expertise, was the reason I suffered this tonic-clonic seizure. And now I sat, six weeks later, uncovering all of this in an old armchair across from Micah. I suppose this new decisive moment can be seen in one of two ways: another random coincidence, or a chance to make a decision that will forever change my story.

I felt insane and didn't care. I sensed, as deeply as I'd known anything, the presence of this attacking tumor on the speech comprehension and creation areas of my brain was designed by God specifically for me. And it was uncovered now for a particular reason. My desire to communicate—to fulfill my life purpose—was so strong I was now willing to lay my life on the line in order to face it.

That was the moment I chose to engage. Difficult decisions immediately became clear, like a haze unexpectedly lifting off my runway. Cancer represented much more than rogue cells multiplying too quickly; it had grown bigger, into a sentient evil agent capable of finding and destroying my very purpose. It was seen as a biological issue in the medical realm, but I felt it was born out of my emotional, mental, and spiritual struggles. I knew exactly how this story would end. I would eliminate this cancer by removing it from my body, either by treatments or by miracles. I would focus my passion on communicating my story with anyone who would listen. If this was indeed my kung fu commission, I wasn't going to waste it. No more running.

There were no words to contain my faith at that moment. It came from an unknown place of divine confidence capable of fueling me to make the biggest decision of my life. My mind turned to Old Testament Bible stories, where characters were asked to make dreadful decisions, to put their life on the line and hope that God would show up. I felt like David stepping forward to hurl a single stone at Goliath. I felt like Moses stepping in front of the pharaoh and demanding freedom for his people. My story paled in comparison to theirs, but maybe this decision was my decision. And if I believed that God and I were indeed on the same writing team, why couldn't I believe He constructed a tedious twenty-seven-year Act I and Act II to perfectly set the stage for this life-changing inciting incident? Accepting this route as my reality actually meant that I could die based on my decision to move forward in faith, but I no longer cared. This was my chance to put pen to paper. This was my chance to tell my story.

Micah opened the door for me that day, but it took several difficult conversations between Amy and I to truly process the ramifications of our next action. We prayed together, on our knees over a tear-stained blue couch, as we chose this road of alternative treatment. Neither of us had any idea what this oncoming battle would require, but I feel absolutely confident that it was a decision made through true and honest faith.

The day before I was to start my radiation treatment, after having been fitted for a mask and learning the procedures of my sessions, I called my doctor at the University of Michigan Cancer Center and told her I was choosing to pass on the conventional treatment of radiation and chemotherapy.

"You are doing *what?* Your radiation starts tomorrow!"

I felt horrible. I hate letting people down and knew this would personally hurt her after she had walked this road with us over the past three weeks. In an attempt to ease the scenario, I used medical terminology to lie to her.

"I know, but I've decided to observe the tumor."

Observing is the final and rarely spoken of treatment option on the short list of surgery, radiation, and chemotherapy. They have to tell you that it's an option, but they never recommend it unless the patient's scenario allows only weeks to live. You only observe if it's obvious you're about to die.

"For how long? If you observe this for six months, it will only continue to grow. If this happens, we might have to potentially increase the intensity of radiation or chemo when it grows."

"I understand this is a risk, but I'm still going to observe it."

I wanted off the phone but knew she had a final trick up her sleeve. Knowing it was coming, I clenched my eyes shut pretending her words wouldn't sting so bad. "David, you know I had cancer in my early twenties. I know it was a different type, but I went through radiation and chemotherapy and, look at me, I'm doing fine! This is your best option! Our team cares about you, and we want to help give you a longer life. This treatment plan isn't a random decision—it's a decision your entire medical team has discussed and agreed upon."

"Thank you. I really do appreciate everyone's hard work, but I still want to observe it."

"David, please don't do this. You are choosing your own death."

I winced as I heard that response. When you had previously placed your life in someone's hands, it's difficult to hear that person raise their voice, begging you to not choose your own death. It's just another person I'm letting down. She explained how my five- to seven-year prognosis would only get worse if I chose not to follow their treatment path. But I chose to remove myself from the fastidious and well-documented results offered in medicine and hand myself over to my God.

I couldn't believe I had come so close to that first treatment. I was 99 percent ready to move forward with pinpointed radiation beams to burn out my brain cells, chemotherapy drugs to flatten my immune system, potential loss of hair, nausea, and struggling to survive for five to seven years. But now, at the last second, Micah introduced me to an answer for that question of *why*. This new hope seemed to perfectly line up with the characters, subplots, and motivations my life was previously searching desperately for. This new direction was Tits and Ass on speed.

Amy and I chose to overcome cancer without the help of conventional treatment. We stood together, not worried about what the doctors would say or how our friends and family would respond. We put our faith in God to heal, to follow alternative treatments, and trusted we would beat the statistical probability of death. We knew we had listened for the direction of God and had chosen, in faith, His thin and rocky path. This would be the beginning of our new story, of following with determined hope a new road leading to a more abundant life.

Nearly two weeks after my life-changing visit with Micah, I returned to his hippie office. I sat below a large diptych painting of Mary, the mother of Jesus and symbol of divine intervention, draped on the wall above his head. She offered me peace as she overheard me telling Micah I'd chosen against the conventional treatments. I wanted to move forward with him, despite having no idea what this parallel reality looked like or what my alternative treatments might consist of.

I asked Micah for my first set of directions. "What next? Where do we begin? Herbal pills? Teas? Do I have to become one of those vegans?"

Micah smiled, filling the room again with his calm presence, and told me we would dive into the details soon. But first, he wanted to warn me of the detoxification process, called the Herxheimer Reaction.

"Wait. Herx-what? What does that mean?"

"It's the official name for a healing crisis. It's when the body detoxifies itself and your symptoms actually increase. You will feel much worse before anything starts to feel better."

In medical terminology, the Herxheimer Reaction made sense to me. I imagined it similar to starting a diet and feeling the misery of detox for a few days, or stopping smoking and dealing with withdrawal. I understood how my body would physically respond to my new treatment. But at that moment, I could never have imagined how I would suffer—emotionally, mentally, spiritually and relationally through my unique healing crisis. Because if I truly knew what would be required of me, I would have stood up and walked out, promising never to return to Eastern Avenue again.

EIGHT
TREATMENTS

IT FEELS LIKE A HANGOVER. The decisions you made last night seemed clear and purposeful and God-given at the time, but now, waking up the day after, you have to deal with the decision you made. Two weeks later, I entered the same back-alley office off Eastern Avenue to see Micah again. This unique individual had completely flipped my decision upside down, from conventional treatments to fighting this cancer naturally. And the only cure for this decision hangover was my Micah-hug that waited patiently for me. This was our official meeting to talk about what would be coming next. And after our typical greetings and polite Q&A, we began.

"First off," he says, "Let me test you."

I had no idea what that meant. He asked me to stand facing him and hold out my right hand in a fist in front of me. He tried to push down on my hand, but I kept it steady where it was. Then he told me to clear my mind as he put a bag of M&M'S in my left hand. Again, he pushed down on my right hand and it sunk. I was shocked to see I couldn't resist his pressure. I told him that wasn't fair because he pushed harder the second time. He denied it and began to explain.

"David, your body is essentially a magnet. You have a positive side, which is your head, and a negative side, which is your feet. I am going to test your body and essentially ask it what it wants or what it needs. When I introduce you to something your body doesn't want, your right hand will dip down because that item is messing with or weakening your body's magnet. Here, try this." He asked me to take my left hand and put my palm on my head. He pushed down on my right hand and it was strong. Then he asked me to turn my left hand over so my palm was facing up. As he pushed, my right hand dipped down. I start laughing, not able to figure out how he is doing this. *Is this actually real?* He explained the hands are a part of these magnetic frequencies as well. So, when the positive side of my hand was on my head, I could resist the pressure. But when the negative palm side of my hand was facing upward, I couldn't resist and showed weakness.

Then he gave me a banana. I put it in my left hand, and with the same pressure, he pushed down on my right hand. Didn't move. He gave me back the M&M'S, pushed down, and I couldn't hold my right hand up. I was in shock! So, then Micah closed his eyes and began repeatedly pushing down on my right hand. Sometimes it would stay up and sometimes it would sink down. "How are you doing this?" I asked in awe. He told me that based on what he was thinking, my body, only being touched by his hand, responded to it. He was thinking through lists of items he had to offer me and my body was responding positively or negatively to them. I was fascinated. As he was doing this, he was taking mental notes about what my body needed. Then he stopped, went over to his products, and started gathering them together on the side table.

In essence, my brain was tallying up an expensive list to reinvigorate my thymus and get my immune system working again. We spent that time putting together a strict vegetarian diet with only a few hints of wild salmon, alongside fruits, lots of vegetables, garlic, seeds, and tons of nuts. He recommended pills such as High Potency Protease, Pau d'arco, silica cell salt, and Pro-Pancreas. He showed me how to apply essential oils such as Frankincense, Three Wise Men®, Thieves®, and Clove®. He showed me how to apply it to my forehead and the bottom of my big toes. He even wanted me to include drops from food-grade hydrogen peroxide into my water as well as drinking small cups of apple cider vinegar each day. No more white flour, pasta, corn, cheese, sugar, alcohol, or coffee. I had already gotten rid of those last two while in the Mayo hospital, but the rest of this list seemed overwhelming.

He introduced me to his kombucha mother, his jellyfish living in a mason jar, and sent me home with a big jar of what looked like a rather nice IPA to drink.

Then he told me I needed to drink ionized, alkalized water because of the higher percentage of oxygen it dumps into your body. He encouraged me to start a regular sauna routine to sweat out the toxins that would be pulled from my body and gave me pills to cleanse the parasites from my digestive tract. He instructed me to watch *The Gerson Therapy*, a documentary discussing how by strictly juicing, cancer can disappear—not *blending*, but actually *juicing* and removing the pulp. He explained that *The Gerson Therapy* consists of drinking thirteen glasses of juice per day while eating as much raw (uncooked food) as possible.

Micah told me the main issue with cancer was centered around the pancreas. According to him, the pancreas represented the core of your inner child. It represented the sweetness of life, but it also pointed at issues of feeling rejected. I was still slowly adapting to this new line of thought, but after coming to grips with the emotional heart lines he previously saw in my eyes, I realized I was already neck deep in it. So, I kept nodding my head, promising to stick with Micah's plan. Whenever I returned to Micah, he honed in on the foods I was eating and showing me how my body was responding. I admit, the time we spent editing my diet was the healthiest I'd ever physically felt.

On one of my visits, Micah recommended another chiropractic doctor in town, Dr. Fan, who also fought cancer through different methods. I had absolutely no idea how a chiropractic doctor could help, but again, I agreed. I called and set up a meeting to see him later in October.

Two months after my diagnosis, Amy and I went to Omaha to attend my ten-year high school reunion as well as share my story for the first time with a local church. I was excited for my high school reunion. But of course, everyone had to welcome me and remind me of my line in *Election*, "What happened to your eye?" I've heard of a lot of bad high school reunion stories, but it was a blast for me. Plus, after following Micah's diet I had lost twenty pounds in a single month. At the reunion I reconnected with people from the marching band, jocks, nerds, actors, everyone. I knew that word had already spread to my class that I was diagnosed with cancer a mere two months earlier. I guess they expected me to be on the brink of death, but I was just as alive, if not more, than I was ten years ago.

On Sunday of that weekend, I showed up to talk at Papillion's Shadow Ridge Church. This was my first time sharing my message, and I was well prepared. I wrote notes on a single piece of paper from my journal with my hit-points and prepared for a half-hour delivery. This was it. This was my first attempt to explain my story to a group of interested people, exactly what I had always wanted to do.

I made sure my talk was packed with humor, shock, and to my surprise, even my own tears. It felt to me as if it was a masterful delivery, but I had no idea what it felt like to the audience.

The main message was that each of us were telling stories with our lives. And when we looked at Hebrews 11, the stories God seems to love the most are the absolutely insane ones. It was in those stories that God showed up and interacted with humanity. But to enter into these stories, each of these Biblical characters had to take a chance, choosing to follow God's small narrow path, to live a life with only a tiny percentage chance of survival. In Hebrews 11:16, God says that those who choose to follow Him down *His* path "desired a better country, that is, a heavenly one. Therefore, God is not ashamed to be called their God, for he has prepared for them a city."

Near the end of my talk, I declared that I chose alternative treatments to follow what I felt God had told me. That in living "our" story and walking down His narrow path, I desired, no matter the outcome, that one day God would tell me He was proud to be called my God. In the end, I put that open question before the audience. When you stand before God in Heaven, will He be proud to be called your God? Will you live that life of faith, even in the worst of times?

My body was on fire during that talk. I wasn't nervous, but my body had been craving the act of telling my story. And afterwards, I had grandmothers, young kids, and parents coming up to me wiping away their tears, profusely thanking me for being there and sharing my story with them. *This is it*, I thought. This is exactly what I was meant to do. Maybe this is how I was created to be "set apart." I was so energized by discovering how my scenario was relating to the audience that I had to have more if it. Speaking had just become a drug to me.

In the next few months, people continued to call me and ask me to visit and speak to their church or university. Every single time, my response was yes. I was still on leave from Dot&Cross, so I was available, and this act of speaking, I realized, was my dream. To share *my* story—not Marcus, Rob, or Josh's—with those who were interested.

My speaking career bloomed over the next few months. I became extremely vocal about my spirituality on my blog, sharing stories, and keeping everyone updated on my progressing health. I had never shared so much about my faith before, but I realized when you are diagnosed with terminal cancer, everyone gives you a free pass to say whatever you want. I felt like I was finally lining up with God's purpose for me and living my dream.

In between these speaking trips, Amy and I always returned home to Grand Rapids. I attended the meeting that Micah had recommend with his friend, Dr. Fan. When I entered, a short Chinese man walked up to shake my hand and performed a small formal bow. He introduced me to his wife behind the counter, who was still learning her English, and his children running around the office who spoke no English at all. I told him my story of learning about this cancer through kung fu and he politely laughed. I told him about the diet changes and essential oils I was now using. He agreed with all of them. Then he escorted me back to one of his rooms and asked me to lie face down on the table.

I had never been to a chiropractic doctor before, but I was familiar with what they do. He did a series of cracks on my spine and, apparently, lengthened one of my legs. It all felt so good, like I was a wooden boy being turned into a real boy. Being unfamiliar with this type of work, I asked him how he knew to do all of this without first doing any type of overview through x-rays of my body or spine.

"It's simple," he said in his thick Chinese accent as he smiled at me. "God shows me."

"What?" I said in shock.

"Yes, God shows me what needs to be done, and then I do that." He was entirely serious. He explained the process to me. He asked the Lord to help him, and one day the Lord started speaking to him and showing him what was wrong, and then he would make the necessary adjustments. To this day I still don't know how he accomplishes it, but I suppose God works with each of us differently. When I desire to speak, God shows up. If Dr. Fan desires to help heal people's backs, God shows up.

Dr. Fan put together an even bigger stack of pills for me than the one Micah had come up with, explained I needed to drink much more water and eat raw calf liver every four hours, and scheduled our next appointment. As I was checking out with his wife at the front of his shop, Dr. Fan picked up a bucket and described the details of performing an enema. Curious about his colorful explanation of how it works, I purchased the unroasted coffee beans and the enema bucket with the intent to start that process of removing parasites from my body.

As I was on my way out the door, he realized he had forgotten to tell me about a book, written by Dr. William D. Kelley. It's called, *Dr. Kelley's Answer to Cancer.* It's all about healing the body through diet, nutritional pills, removing toxins through enemas and sweating, and replacing lost enzymes in the pancreas via "Pan-alone" pills that fight cancer in the body. I read on the back of the book that Dr. Kelley had been doing research on cancer patients for some time, but when he learned he had pancreatic cancer, the worst of them all, he dedicated himself to finding *the answer to cancer*. This story had to be complete malarkey, like it was being sold on a Saturday morning telethon. But the front of the book proclaimed Dr. Kelley's confidence by saying he had "cured tens of thousands of people from cancer." I felt I owed it to Dr. Fan to buy the book and promised him I would read it.

I had a strange dream that night after picking up my pills and enema supplies. Of course, dreams had taken on an entirely new significance to me since Amy had begun digging deep into books regarding dreams as signs from God. She explained to me that colors represented specific things, and even traveling in specific dream vehicles can carry divine symbolism. But in my dream, I was in an airport and walking to my gate to wait for the plane to depart. There were two guys at the gate also waiting to board the same plane. Oddly enough, they were dressed in karate uniforms (or "Gi"), which are the typical baggy, white karate outfits with the signature thick belts tied around the waist.

These two men approached me and kindly, yet bluntly, told me they believed in the power of healing and asked if they could pray for me. I quickly agreed, knowing full-well you do whatever kung fu experts tell you to do. Each of them put one hand on my shoulder and one hand on my back. Feeling somewhat silly for taking these kind gentlemen's time, I stopped them and said, *"Um, if you are going to pray for my healing, you should know that I have a brain tumor. Maybe you could pray specifically for that."* Quietly, they removed their hands from my shoulders and put their hands on my head and neck. They began praying silently, and I could feel a great peace come over my body. It was such a comforting feeling. The two guys took their hands off my head and neck and looked at each other as though they had both encountered the same type of mutual understanding regarding my cancer. Then, simultaneously, they both looked at me. When they did, I completely understood two specific things:

1. I understood they both knew what was going to happen to me. They didn't hint that I would be healed or that I would die, but it was certain they both knew the final outcome of this brain tumor.

2. I understood that I could not ask them the outcome. Even if I did ask, they were not going to tell me.

And then I woke up.

A few weeks later, we got a call from Jasmine and J.D. Star. They told us that we should all take a trip together and we got to choose the location.

I remembered what I had told the nurse as she put on my mask before my surgery. I didn't want to go to Tokyo, but rather to New Zealand. We threw the idea out there and they agreed. So, we pulled together what money we had, and Jasmine and J.D. helped with the remaining funds. Then, in the days after Christmas, we hopped on a plane headed for Christchurch, New Zealand.

The trip, both in sights and in stories, was ridiculous. We shared stories of our families, the photography world, and the plan Amy and I had made to deal with my cancer. We spent New Year's Eve in Queenstown, New Zealand, on the Southern landmass. After allowing a temporary pass on my diet, we all sat around and gorged ourselves on incredible food as we sat in a second-story restaurant overlooking Lake Wakatipu. I realized that New Zealand was the furthest country to the east and would be the first to see the sun in this new year. So, I tried, with all I had, to convince my travel partners to stay up all night to drive to the beach and to be some of the first humans to see the sun rise in the year 2010. And for quite good reasons (namely my health), I lost that battle. But we did stay at our restaurant through the entire night, overlooking a mass of people at a public dance party in the streets. I remember the gentleman who climbed up on a post at the edge of the dock, taller than everyone dancing their hearts out. And when that clock struck midnight, with ancient bells echoing out over the entire town, he did a full backflip fifteen feet above, what I imagined to be, freezing cold water. Everyone went absolutely nuts and screamed (of course with the New Zealand accent).

On December 31st in Queenstown, New Zealand, on the last day of 2009—the year I heard the worst news of my life—Amy and I were celebrating with some of our best friends in one of my favorite new locations. We loved our food, drinks, and conversation as we celebrated a new year inside that beautiful city tucked between gorgeous mountains. We were able to turn our heads and gaze out over the water until it all disappeared into fog. The sites, the people, and the feelings of that single New Year's Eve, easily climbed the list to make it one of the top ten moments of my life.

Several days later, on our scenic drive back to Christchurch for our flight home, Amy and I arrived to spend a day at a small beachside town named Kaikoura. We took a long walk up the beach where I witnessed a landscape I will never forget. I looked to the right at this beautifully clean and dark blue ocean bringing in massive rolling waves. The crashing, furious water shot enough mist into the air to catch the sunlight and form rainbows. Watching these waves envelop each other was breathtaking. The water gathered itself, sneaking up onto a mystical black-sand beach—where the deeper you dug, the blacker the sand appeared— then retreating just as quickly back into the ocean. Then looking to the left, the beach gave way to a fenced-in area that housed goats and sheep bleating away their afternoon. And just beyond this open field was an incredibly large rugged mountain range with snow still on its caps.

If an alien were to visit earth, I would tell them to go down to the beach and watch as Nature shows off everything she's got, and then I'd tell them to buy a fridge magnet and take it back to their home planet. This was a view I wanted my life to be filled with: My beautiful Amy and I standing barefoot on a once-in-a-lifetime beach on the other side of the world. Somewhere back in Michigan, life was moving on, photos of kids were being taken, and films were being made. But not here, not now. To us, Kaikoura, New Zealand was God's own version of heaven on earth.

NINE
JOURNEY TO JAMAA

EVERY GREAT VACATION COMES SCREECHING TO AN END when reality smacks you in the face. When we returned to Grand Rapids, it was time to get back to work. Having taken a long break from Dot&Cross, I was ready to re-engage with my life. I made all the necessary changes to my diet, starting drinking specific kinds of tea, and taking my 150 pills per day. Dr. Fan was quite specific when he explained to me how to properly perform an enema. I was to take two tablespoons of unroasted coffee and mix it with a liter of water, heat it to a boil on the stove, then let it sit on low heat for twenty minutes. It came out steaming hot, so I had to let it sit for an hour or so before it cooled to the right temperature.

Next, I poured the liquid, too light in color to properly be called coffee, into my enema bucket and hung it on the door handle of the guest room. I was to lie on my side on the floor and place the long tube next to my nether regions. Then I would take the red part of the tube (a foot and a half in length) and prepare it for insertion. Of course, this extra-long tube was Dr. Fan's own modification. These enema buckets typically came with a short insertion attachment of 1 or 2 inches, but that didn't fit his standards for a proper enema. So, he found an 18-inch replacement to offer his clients. I used the oil olive to grease it up, and in the quiet of our bedroom, I inserted it.

Of course, this felt quite strange. I released the plastic tube blocker allowing the water to flow through. HOLY SHIT, TOO HOT! I had no idea what the proper temperature of coffee was for the inside of my ass, but this was way too hot for me.

I lay there for another twenty minutes, scared to take out the tube and replace it. But finally it cooled off, and I released the coffee again. Thankfully, it wasn't nearly as hot this time. I could feel the coffee entering and essentially, filling me up from the opposite direction. About one third of the way through the bucket, I realized I was about to explode. I was stopping the liquid every few seconds to let my insides recover. But now, I felt I couldn't hold it any longer. Quickly, I reset the plastic blocker, removed the enema bucket from the doorknob, and ran for the bathroom. I barely made it. I'll leave out the details, but just imagine your cluttered basement, filled with junk you know you'll never actually need, being completely cleaned out in about ten seconds. It was a holy experience.

I went back to finish off the final two-thirds and, once again, ran back to the bathroom. I know how weird this sounds, but there are few things more pleasurable in life that emptying your bowels after an enema. I could give you a list of the fancy people in my life who I've convinced to perform these same enemas, but releasing that list would be the final thing I would do for them.

I continued doing this twice a day, every day. Once in the morning and again in the late afternoon. It was a great replacement for drinking coffee because the caffeine absorbed into my system so quickly that it woke me up immediately. And when performed on a regular basis, I would start passing all sorts of parasites. And by parasites, I mean clumps of long stringy things, including nests for future generations of parasites that have invaded my body against my will. They were living in my digestive system and were removing the nutrition from my food for themselves before my body could absorb it.

It took time, but eventually I got to the point where I could hold two complete buckets (nearly 100 ounces) in my gut. My body was so clean I lost cravings for sugar, slept better, and digested food better. It was amazing. So, I took it everywhere with me. To make that happen I bought a camping percolator. All I had to do was plug it in and turn it on. It became my travel staple. And the best part was that airport security had no idea what to do with this. Ninety percent of the time, I was called out of the line so security could search my bag. I had a mason jar filled with uncooked coffee grounds, a long tube, and my camping percolator. I can only imagine this series of strange contraptions must have looked exactly like a bomb. Eventually, getting called out of line and searched for each and every flight became very annoying. I started out by announcing, even before going through security, that I had a percolator in my bag, but still they searched me. In fact, I was so frustrated that I decided to create an enjoyable experience out of the process. I decided to just give the unfiltered and louder than normal truth to any TSA agent who handled the tube: "That's the part I stick up my ass!" That usually got things moving.

Next, my wife and I purchased the Norwalk Juicer featured in the Gerson Treatment film. It was a beast of a machine. It cost a ridiculous amount of money, and the process of juicing took a horrendous amount of time. The original idea of juicing thirteen times per day became a joke. People told me I could juice once in the morning then store it, but every article I read talked about how much nutrition is lost, per second, when the juice is stored. And I, a nutritional moron, was still eager enough to pursue perfection.

First, you put the fruit or vegetable in a loud spinning chopper (a triturator) that mashes it into a wet cloth. Now the food is chunky and juicy. Then you take this cloth and place it on a hydraulic press that slowly compresses the food as the juice runs out of it. The amount of pressure this machine creates is insane, which is probably why it weighs as much as it does. Amy and I began planning for as many juices as we could muster in a single day.

We would wash, peel, mash, squeeze, clean. Wash, peel, mash, squeeze, clean. The whole process, start to finish, took about forty minutes per juice. For each juice, we would use enough greens to make two to three salads: kale, spinach, and Swiss chard (essentially the darkest greens available). At first, I tried to make things taste good. I would add a piece of fruit or a hint of ginger or coconut water. But after a few weeks, I gave up on taste. When you are juicing to save your life, taste goes out the window.

When I determined to take part in Dr. Kelley's treatment, it was financially intense. Dot&Cross paid me a substantial amount of money, and Amy made even more than I did. We were definitely privileged D.I.N.K.S. (Double Income No Kids), but instead of shopping or going on vacations, we bought pills. It cost us about $2,500 a month to buy all of the pills Dr. Fan recommended. I started out with Dr. Kelley's pills, the most expensive, set on reestablishing the proper activity of my pancreas. We also purchased the rest of Dr. Fan's recommendations and Micah's nutritional vitamins and oils as well.

I started taking 150 pills per day. The point was to get my barely working pancreas to start producing the right enzymes to fight cancer within my body. Of course, no medical doctor would ever prescribe this, and my insurance company laughed in my face when I brought it up. I chose not to follow the path of conventional medicine, the chemotherapy and the radiation that fries your body, in order to take this alternative route, which would end up taking half our money and half of our time. We were certain this was the path that was needed in order for God to heal me.

In addition to the enemas, diet, and pills, I was also dedicated to sitting in a sauna for two hours a day. Dr. Fan gave me instructions for how to build an indoor sauna, and I had my brother-in-law, Jonathan, come over and build it in our guest bedroom. I'd completely given up on the idea of ever building anything myself, so Jon saved the day.

My new morning routine would be to wake up early, perform a half-hour enema, sit in the sauna for forty-five minutes as sweat poured from my body, take about twenty pills, shower, then juice for forty-five minutes. Each morning I performed this two- to three-hour routine.

But that wasn't it. I had to complete that same process in the afternoon after my vegan lunch had completely digested. Again, I would perform an enema, take more pills, sit in the sauna, shower, and juice. All day long I would be taking twenty pills every four hours till I went to sleep. It became so rote that my life turned into a manufacturing line. I had no time to see, let alone hang out with my friends. And even if I did, I couldn't enjoy a beer or some hot wings. As an extrovert, this cleansing process was killing my soul, while apparently restoring my body. Always seems to be one or the other, doesn't it?

I moved from our loud and overwhelming group office to a much smaller single-room office down the street, upstairs from our world-renowned HopCat Brewery. I set up my green writing desk and brought in a chair from home. I worked from there but felt like things still weren't the same. When everything else in life feels off kilter, I return to my mental basecamp and start digging through my Bible. I would work for maybe half a day, then spend the rest of the day reading about Old Testament characters and taking comfort in their completely ridiculous and overwhelming stories.

This new search seemed to both help and frustrate me at the same time. Amy had been bothering me about my lack of spirituality. In college, she dumped me for a week because I didn't speak in tongues as the Bible described. It wasn't that I was opposed to it, it just seemed like a something a religious zealot would convince you was required. Wanting to both please my wife while also pursuing God, I determined that I was going to continue to press on God until He showed me the details of this gift. Wanting desperately to be healed, I was open to anything, even speaking in tongues. But I didn't want some three-piece-suit pastor laying his hands on me and screaming at me in the middle of a church worship riot. I wanted this for myself, knowing full well it was God who gave this gift.

I sat in my office, digging through Jack Deere's book, *Surprised by the Power of the Spirit*. I would sit in deep prayer, honestly crying out, begging for God to deliver me the gift of spiritual tongues. Considering the fact that worship music sucks today, I went back to the same Keith Green album, *For Him Who Has Ears To Hear*, over and over again. I read through his book, *No Compromise*, then read another book, *A Heavenly Man*, by Brother Yun, about his escapades in China involving the Holy Spirit. I worshipped the Lord, sang through the songs that connected with me as I drew closer to Him. Day after day, I would go through this. And one day, after hours and hours, wiping away my own frustrated tears, I stopped trying and told the Lord it was up to him. I couldn't fabricate this spiritual manifestation.

On my knees in my office, crying and praising, weeping and practically yelling, my energy level started increasing. My oneness with God started to overlap my physical reality. I didn't feel alone anymore. Crouched on the floor I felt as though I was surrounded by electricity filling up my body as I experienced what seemed to be a spiritual orgasm. Then an unknown language started rolling off my lips.

At first, I couldn't believe it and thought I had fooled myself into this. But immediately, I felt the Holy Spirit come over me and an overwhelming sense of peace and comfort. All of my slamming, banging, and punching on God's front door, had finally found its relief when God opened it. I sat there and prayed in tongues for the rest of the afternoon, this strange, heavenly language moving easily from my lips. Despite the times I had tried in the past to "instruct" these words to exit, they now flowed smoothly out of my mouth.

But from that moment on, whenever I run out of words to say or whenever I need to pray for someone but have no idea what to pray for, I speak in tongues. And each and every time, the peace of God flows over me. I admit, it is a bizarre way to pray. And I, the one who demands scientific results for nearly everything I do, simply can't explain it. But I also can't deny its effect on me when I finally felt heard by God.

One day I got word that World Vision was going to shoot a narrative movie in Uganda. I contacted my old college roommate, Jon Brown, a World Vision employee working on similar projects, who gave me the right numbers to call. After talking to them about the future of this project, we realized the production budget wouldn't be near what Dot&Cross would require, but we could gladly offer our services as film consultants. I proposed our offer and World Vision agreed. In early 2010, I began preparing for my trip to Uganda in March.

In preparation for our trip, I was told I needed inoculations to cover the barrage of diseases that were alive and flourishing in Uganda. But the last thing I wanted to do was to put more toxic junk into my body. So, before we left, I called Bob Goff, my friend who had somehow become a consul for the country of Uganda. I asked if he would send me an official Ugandan letter saying I was exempt from the border patrol restrictions and must be let into the country. And should I encounter any problems, he typed his phone number into the document and would be standing by to answer. It's moments like this when I still can't believe the way that God has worked Bob into my life.

I had no idea what to expect. This was my first trip to sub-Saharan Africa. So, I bought outdoor clothes that didn't need washing and purchased an Indiana Jones hat, knowing one day I'd use it as my memoir of the trip. The day came when I flew to Amsterdam to meet my team before we all flew to Uganda together. I met the film's director, Michael Landon Jr. (son of Michael Landon of *Little House on the Prairie* and *Bonanza* fame), and a writer, Brian Bird, who since has gone on to find great success in Hollywood.

We arrived at Ugandan customs, and as everyone was handing over their passports, their luggage would be briefly inspected. I handed over my passport and my letter from Bob. The customs workers looked at it vexed, as if this letter were some anomaly. Then he felt for the raised stamp of the Ugandan flag in the corner, shrugged, and allowed me to come through. It's good to have friends in high places.

We got in the vans and left for our hotel. My bag was filled to the brim with pills and enema supplies. It was shocking to drive past homes of people who had absolutely no money, while in my bag were ten days' worth of pills equal in dollars to their yearly income. I felt guilty for being born in the United States and actually being offered a fighting chance at defeating this cancer.

Our hotel was mediocre, and the hanging mosquito nets over our beds reminded us what we were in for. I woke up the next morning determined to be dedicated and maintain my routine, so I heated up my coffee enema water and took my morning horse pills with my bottled water. The bathroom was sticky with heat, so I threw down towels to lie on as I performed my enema while listening to mosquitos buzzing all around me. These malaria infested demons had overrun the country, and I prayed to God not to get bitten.

A few nights into this project, I heard there was a Bible-based healer coming through town. As always, I was quite leery but wanted to experience what was happening. After a full day of working, I took Barry, a World Vision employee with whom I'd made friends, with me. We went into a crowd of nearly two thousand people gathered around a massive stage in a giant field. And just as I imagined, the African equivalent of Benny Hinn came on stage and began speaking in Ugandan. Barry and I were standing near the back, taking it all in. As the voices of the crowd increased, it started getting raucous. But Barry and I witnessed an elderly woman, unable to walk, get wheeled onto the stage. After being prayed for, she got up and started walking, or more so stumbling, across the rest of the stage as she laughed and cried. Men, blind for their whole lives, could finally turn their gaze to see the stage lights and see their family members for the first time. A group of ten men who had never heard a single sound began weeping as they started hearing the crowd singing to them. The place was going absolutely bananas for God and His healing powers.

A large part of me wanted to step on that stage with the expectation that I would be healed of cancer. When God healed, He healed, regardless of what language was being spoken. But I was too shy. I knew I would be so out of place. My tears moved from joy to disappointment and fear. Barry saw my agony, and he put his arm around my shoulder knowing exactly what I was thinking. I just stood there in the back and cried at the miracles being performed in front of me, while distinctly choosing not to step forward. I even prayed in tongues, searching for an answer as to what to do next. Was this the moment God had set aside for me? To be healed in a nation where it seems to happen constantly? Like in that book, *A Heavenly Man*, where God would, on the spot, continually heal people whose hearts have not become dull to His Spirit.

I will never know if that moment was meant for me and was so disappointed I never even tried.

As far as the actual project, we ended up putting together a script based on the true story of two kids whose mother died of Malaria. They packed her body in a coffin, put that coffin on wheels, and managed to walk it through Kampala to their

Aunt's house two full days away. When they arrived, the uncle, who was already overwhelmed with the number of his own children, was concerned about adding two more kids to their family. In the night, the two children heard the arguments over whether or not their aunt and uncle could provide food for them, so in the morning they snuck out, having nowhere to go and no source of income. When their aunt realized they had left, she went out to search for them, found them on the side of a busy road, and brought them back home to their family.

Michael, Brian, and I began scripting out their story based on their retellings. And through our translators, we came up with the idea of naming this film *Journey to Jamaa*. Jamaa is a Ugandan word that translates to "eternal family."

I returned home from Uganda on March 30th. My company was a mess. I had changed offices, Sonny and Corey had moved to Los Angeles, but the ongoing Dot&Cross problems had found me and were starting to turn sour. We were struggling to stay on the same page, and each of our new projects seemed to be leading each of us in different directions.

During that same time period, Amy had turned a unique spiritual corner. She told me that God had given her dreams about how close the end of America was. She even told me the specific dates when this would start to happen. She explained that in the next year or two, we would see another economic crash, so we needed to start storing up food. She went into detail regarding an oncoming earthquake on the New Madrid Fault Line that would cause a 100-foot tidal wave to hit and destroy Chicago. It would go on to flood the Missouri River covering entire states, essentially wiping out the Midwest. Then the damaged United States was to be taken over by Russian and Japanese armies. Americans, but more importantly *Christian* Americans, will be persecuted and put into re-education camps.

Then a few days later, she told me of another dream featuring Burl Ives singing "Silver and Gold." She saw that as a prophetic dream telling her we needed to purchase silver in order to avoid the upcoming crash of the dollar. She explained the investment opportunity and how silver would outlast the failing dollar (which actually sounded pretty solid to me following 2008's crash). I didn't necessarily disagree with this, so we ended up buying over $10,000 worth of silver bullion (silver bars). And when they arrived, weighing nearly a ton, I carried them up our stairs and put that giant box into our hall closet. Then we covered them up with gloves and hats as our greatest investment sat warm beneath our winter clothes.

Then came another dream. Amy told me my cancer would be healed in August of 2010. Strangely enough, I learned Dr. Fan had a similar dream as well. Not to mention that Dr. Fan's wife had recently told me through her broken English that she had a dream that said I would be soon opening presents, like it was my birthday. She told me through her smile and broken English that God was going to heal me.

Amy had convinced me that Dr. Fan and her dreams were a message from God about my healing. Knowing that Amy was closer to God than I was, I trusted her and stepped up to tell Dr. Fan, in faith, I would stop purchasing the expensive Pan-alone pills. We believed that in August, God was going to show up and heal my brain cancer. I stayed true to our plan, spending what spare moments I had in our guest room sauna, emptying my coffee-filled bowels, throwing back my massive stack of pills, downing my fifth juice every day, and praying the MRI that I would take in August would be the last I ever needed because my brain would be completely restored. I was physically and spiritually putting myself on the line.

But everything else in life was a mess. Dot&Cross was disintegrating before my eyes, and all I heard from Amy were prophecies about earthquakes, floods, and foreign takeovers. The only thing I had to hold onto was this prophecy that I would soon be healed. When considering all of this, it actually started to make sense. I had heard and seen enough stories to know that when life starts to truly fall apart, expect to see another miracle from God.

So, August 2010 became my deadline. I placed my undivided hope in God to be miraculously healed of cancer. I wanted my life to serve as a signpost that God still exists and He still performs miracles on behalf of those who place their complete trust in Him. I wanted to add my story as evidence, displaying what happens when I focus on moving forward with nothing but deep faith that God can and will heal me.

Please, dear God, please show up.

I was overwhelmed. I was in the middle of the massive consultation with World Vision that I was attempting to finish on my own. Sonny and Corey (half of Dot&Cross) had moved to Los Angeles, which divided our resources, slowly pulling our company apart, and not providing us enough income to pay our ten employees. So, Brett had to start letting them go. This was miserable because we had built up such a great team, including my brother-in-law, Michael. In addition, we had to let go of my close friends, Aaron and Sue. We also had to let go of Seth and Sally, who both worked for us and were also married. Meanwhile, at home my wife was explaining, in great prophetic detail, the end of America.

TEN
SECRET SINS

IT WAS TIME FOR A SPIRITUAL OVERHAUL. Having been upended by Uganda's conditions, seeing the movements of God I witnessed, and hearing Amy's ongoing prophecies of healing, I became rampant in my studying of God's Word, as well as additional study books and prayer guides. I wrote and wrote in my journals about my sin as I sought forgiveness. Despite what was clear and obvious about the reality of my illness, I kept praying that I would be completely and 100 percent healed in August. But honestly, I was turning into a mess.

My journal entries seemed bipolar. One day I was eager to learn and heal, but the next day I'd be lazy, attempting to pull myself out of the bed. Full of the Spirit one day and doubting the next. It seems these extreme differences I was going through were evidence of what was going on in my life. My treatments allowed no time to be spent with friends, no hobbies, and limited time to work each day. No more wine or cheese. No more meat. No more cold beers on the porch. It seemed like all of life's best tiny moments were taken from me and replaced by a naturopathic anvil I had to carry.

It took nothing for me to break my diet. Any excuse would do. Well, tonight is so-and-so's birthday. Well, tonight let's celebrate a new project I recently finished.

My attitude toward my health sucked, and my daily habits were even worse. I repeatedly went to the Lord asking for motivation, inspiration, creativity, and wisdom, but received nothing in return. In a moment to shock God with my faith, Amy and I chose a date for my healing in August and prayed like mad to be healed on that date, until it came and went. Like a thrashing child, I could only hope that God was just sitting, holding me, waiting for me to wear myself out.

I wasn't feeling "set apart" at all. Maybe "left outside" is better phraseology. I felt like an add-on for Dot&Cross in our final projects together. I had developed a new company, RobinHood Ink., that was brewing and waiting in the wings. But the attempt to balance each of my projects and my insane life left me writing new prescriptions for myself every day in my journal. No more alcohol. Only one movie per week. Pursue weekly scheduled interactions with friends. Daily prayers. But all of this caused me to nearly give up on everything and accept a boring, frustrating This and That life. I kept telling God how badly I needed him and that I was sick of His silence.

The only thing that brought me up from this rubble was the opportunity to share my story. A chance to climb up out of my hole and see actual people, to pray with people, to make people laugh, to make people cry. I knew that was the perfect life for me, and it became the only thing I was holding onto during those days. But otherwise, things kept getting worse. In July, my second mother, Marilyn Amstutz, the first person to visit me in the hospital, learned she had aggressive breast cancer. She would soon be undergoing a double mastectomy. And a few months later, I decided I had to leave Dot&Cross, previously my personal savior. Now I had to rely on my own start-up company, RobinHood Ink.

Amy was told by God I had hidden sins in my life that I was choosing not to ask forgiveness from her for. Being slightly pissed at God, I hated to admit she was right. I knew it was time to spill it. When we were in college, we had dated for a full year when Amy told me she was having serious trouble being with someone who didn't believe in speaking in tongues. She was concerned about me entering Heaven because she then believed that only those who speak in tongues can enter Heaven. She religiously dumped me in a Starbucks café in a Barnes & Noble. I was livid. On my way back home, I called my older sister Angie and angrily yelled through the retelling of this story, of how this wasn't right, of how she didn't see the bigger picture.

The next night I found myself, no…I placed myself at another girl's house. Her name was Ivana, she was from Croatia, and upon her arrival at Cedarville

University, she quickly became the international woman of mystery. She was gorgeous and seemed to rarely play by the rules. She told stories of her days as a Croatian Judo champion as well as being a car-bomb survivor. I remember seeing her walk around campus by herself: incredibly intimidating. I watched people avoid her and glance in opposite directions. But pre-Amy, I determined she would be mine. I was in full pursuit, but for whatever reason, we could never really work out our situation. I still had no idea what I was doing wrong, but none of my moves worked. I tried for months but was only met by her smirk and Dracula accent. But when Amy showed up and we started dating, Ivana got more aggressive. She knew she had previously had me in her pocket, but now I had moved on.

I picked Ivana up, and we went to Dino's coffee shop in Yellow Springs where I told her about the breakup between Amy and I. Essentially, I was telling her the time is now if she wanted to make a move. And she did. After returning from our long conversation we ended up in her driveway making out in my car. Then later that week, we made out again in her kitchen. It was strangely different, but it was strangely good. Still I knew, deep down, I was filling an Amy-shaped hole.

And sure enough, Amy showed up one week later. She walked into my apartment, and I hopped up off the couch, meeting her halfway to embrace her. She told me she didn't know what the answer was but that we would figure it out together. Those were the perfect words to my soul. Of course, we would start dating again. But secretly, that meant I had to steer clear from Ivana, this beautifully rowdy, dark-haired woman who now knew exactly whom she wanted. Even later, while Amy and I were dating, Ivana confronted me, essentially asking me to make a clear decision to choose her over Amy. I hesitantly kissed her again when we went on Thanksgiving break to Philadelphia, but it was so different now that I was dating Amy again. And that was the moment I had "officially" cheated by kissing Ivana while Amy and I were together.

I told Amy all of this and to my surprise, she was filled with amazing grace. I told her of how I needed something at that time. Of how I was angry about our breakup and had to fill what she took from me. I told her that that was the only secret I ever kept from her. But now, coming clean, she seemed okay with my horrible mistake. I was actually in shock over her reaction. Dealing with these issues seemed key because I knew I needed to rid myself of all of my secret sins in order to be healed by the Lord in August of that year. And it seemed that if I had not asked for forgiveness regarding those previous issues, I would be holding back my own healing.

In order to prepare for my miraculous healing, Amy was told by God to ask me if I had ever slept with anyone else during our marriage. Ha! Of course not! I knew I had never cheated on her during our marriage.

But she was certain the Lord had told her I had an affair with another woman. She seemed so certain, declaring that God had told her this specifically, that I actually started to worry. *Had I?* Maybe there was one night on the road when something went horribly wrong? Maybe I was so ashamed of it that I had literally forgotten about it. I was scared at the concept of opening up my mind to rediscover it. I know I had just seen her grace over the previous issue. Would she show me that grace again if I were to admit to this?

To a degree, I almost wish I had slept with someone else. Because then when I came clean about it, there was a chance our relationship could be healed. But still, even in the deepest searches of my memory, her conviction of guilt fell upon an acquitted soul. It felt on a spiritual level that we were on different pages, maybe even different testaments. We needed to find some level ground to meet on.

In the middle of the summer of 2010, I finally witnessed a miracle. Amy came home from the beach telling me she had found a church for us to attend. I was thrilled to hear this because Amy had such a ridiculously high standard of what a church should be. I believed we'd never find a church to attend. She was on the beach with her sister discussing our ongoing situation with my cancer, and a random woman came over to talk to them. Amy explained the nature of my cancer with her and this new woman explained she was the pastor of Regeneration Church in Jenison, about twenty minutes away from our home. The church was Pentecostal, and it preached healing. Many people had been healed in their congregation, and if Amy felt this strongly about us attending this church, I was in!

Before we attended the church, Amy invited the pastor, Tina, and her husband Scott (her co-pastor), over for dinner. That night, I watched as two individuals entered our home that made the hairs on the back of my neck stand on end. My stomach dropped and my feet started tingling. I couldn't tell what, but I got the sense that there was something off with these two people. But I bolstered myself. After my experience in Uganda, after Amy's forgiveness regarding Ivana, was I actually going to say no to the people of God when they show up at my doorstep? I put away my gut feelings and welcomed them to our table. We shared a lovely meal and told them we were looking forward to attending their church on Sunday morning.

After a full year of living with this cancer, I was thrilled to have finally found a church my wife trusted. We drove to Jenison and found ourselves pulling up to a daycare center where the church was currently meeting. We knew it was a start-up church, but had absolutely no idea what we'd find there. When we entered, there was a sparse congregation of only twelve people, and Tina and Scott were at the front waving palm branches in the air.

My guard remained up, but after recent lessons, I knew God worked through strange people in strange places. I wasn't going to miss out on whatever was happening here. We sat through the service, but when I looked at the other attendees in the room, I noticed that each of the women wore a head covering. Again, I refused to jump to any conclusions. I wanted to remain open. I wanted to be completely dedicated to fully taking all of this in.

While sitting there, I felt like this experience was very similar to an excited group of teenagers at a Bible camp. Tina and Scott's young daughter, maybe twelve or thirteen, led the music, and the pastors spoke of their time in Chicago, training to lead this church and how God was constantly telling them to go do this or that. They kept making these grandiose prophecies, telling people they would soon be rich, telling people they were now healed, or set free from demonic spirits, when obviously they weren't. But if you disagreed with these two pastors by saying, "Actually, I'm not healed," you were siding with the enemy which was a serious offense against them and God.

This continued week after week. Amy relished every word as though it were coming from the mouth of God Himself. I felt my soul waving red flags, shooting off flare guns, lighting entire endangered forests on fire, but I wanted to trust Amy so badly. If she was seeing value here, then I told myself I could too. This was all new to me, which meant I just needed to stretch my mind open a little more.

About a month into it, we invited our friends Ryan and Jenny Duffy to come. They were frustrated at their church and needed something different and fresh. But again, that next Sunday with Ryan and Jenny there, despite what was being said or felt or experienced, I felt little to no presence of God in the room. I thought maybe this was my fault. Maybe it was me who was holding back these feelings based on my background of strict religiosity. So, I continued to keep my mouth shut and returned week after week. "God, I'm so confused," I would pray as we drove to Jenison, "Please show up today. Let me see what they are seeing. Let me experience what they are experiencing. Please, God!"

Eventually, after Tina and Scott learned more about me, they called me aside after church one day and asked me to stop traveling and sharing my story. They said I should stop speaking until I'm fully healed. That sounded strange coming from them. They were asking me to stop sharing the only real story I had in my life. A story that, according to reports from the places I was speaking at, was having a serious impact on congregations. I was absolutely certain the point of me speaking wasn't the fact that I *had* been healed, but that I was placing my faith in my God to heal me *in the future*. Tina and Scott strongly disagreed, but it wasn't until Amy agreed with them that I felt the first true shift between us. Something strange was starting to happen.

I had one more previously scheduled speaking event left; my biggest, highest profile speech at Story Conference in Chicago. A few months earlier, Ben Arment called me out of the blue saying he was moved by my blog and asked if I would share my story. I was pleased to. Amy, Ryan, and Jenny all came with me to Chicago and sat in the first few rows as I stood to speak and, once again, cried my way through the second half of my talk. I remember feeling so alive to this group of artists, filmmakers, musicians, writers, speakers, who were all hearing my story for the first time. Tons of people came up to me afterwards, sharing how much they were moved by my story of faith and my hope in God. This was what I ached for while sitting in Micah's office one year earlier. But nevertheless, I had to return home to Michigan, and attend the craziness of Regeneration Church.

The next week, when Amy and I went back into church, Tina declared, "The Lord told me he wants to heal us of our iniquities. If you need healing, come to the front!" I knew what this meant. I overlooked my strong desires to run out the backdoor and instead, asked the Lord for more humility, telling Him I was honestly open to whatever he wanted to do. I went forward. In fact, half of the audience went forward, leaving six up front and six in the audience. In the line of people, Amy stood next to me. I was so confused about what was about to happen. She was weeping and obviously moved by the Spirit of God. I wasn't feeling anything. Maybe I wasn't sure what the Spirit of God actually felt like?

No. I determined that wasn't the case with me. I refused to believe I was incapable of interactions with God. I had been through many spiritual moments in my life, knew I had felt the Spirit of God in me, knew He had moved through me to reach others, and knew His words when spoken in my ear. I knew what it was like to experience God, but this service was nothing like any of that. This church was the equivalent of pitiful mimes attempting a Shakespearean play.

Tina moved down the row as people were being slain in the spirit, falling over to those catching them. I asked God to do as He wanted with me, that I promised I was not going to stand in opposition to whatever He wanted to do, whether or not I liked how it was delivered. And when Tina stood in front of me, my eyes were closed and my heart was open to what the Spirit of the Lord wanted to do. She gave me a slight push to slay me in the spirit. But I felt nothing. I didn't go down at all. I just stood there, thinking maybe I should just go down to save both of us from this awkwardness.

I looked over to see my wife was sprawled out on the floor with a big grin on her face, and as much as I wanted to be knocked over by the Spirit of God, I wasn't. I had previously pursued God to speak in tongues and that had happened, so why did I feel He was leaving me high and dry now?

At the end of the service, Tina approached me, and we had a short conversation about what it means to be slain in the spirit. She asked why I didn't fall. I told her it was because nothing actually happened to me. I feel like it should be something God does as opposed to me just choosing to fall over. I told her I still wanted to participate and was open to these new experiences, but for whatever reason, this wasn't the week for me.

This happened several more times, and I was getting more and more frustrated with this entire scenario. On the day Amy and I had declared I would be healed, the pastors were rather direct and asked me to lie flat on the ground and had four people surround me. I lay down and my face was quite close to the sandals of a man from which rose a horrendous stench. I thought to myself: *David, this is it. Here I am. I am at my lowest point, smelling foot fungus, yet still my heart and my mind are open to allow God to heal me. I am lying prostrate on the ground, regardless of the fact that a child, a teenager, and two grown adults are currently climbing all over my body. This is perfect. When I feel the furthest from myself, from my pride, that is the moment when the spirit of the Lord will know I'm open to His healing.*

So, I stayed on the ground and begged the Lord not to heal me but to just show up and convince me He was nearby.

But again, nothing happened.

Did I still have more secret sins I was hiding? I had told Amy about Ivana. I had confessed to my college professors that I cheated or I was bitter at them. I didn't drink until I was twenty-one. I'd never smoked pot. I didn't have sex until marriage. I never even had a broken bone or a cavity. That was everything I knew! I prayed: *Are there more rules I've broken? More things I haven't confessed? Please show me my unconfessed sins, because it appears I'm not fully ready for the Lord to heal me. I want to be "set apart" and no longer "left outside." I desperately want to be free from this cancer. God, I so badly want to share our story of how you healed me from this inoperable brain tumor, so please, let me be used by you. Let me share this story with the world. Please God, do it now!*

ELEVEN
DEGENERATION CHURCH

TINA AND SCOTT KNEW that Ryan and I were preparing to march up and nail our *95 Theses* to the front door of their childcare center, so they invited our families to dinner at their house. It was a pleasant place in Jenison, but upon arriving, I was shocked to find I was being served by Julia, a quiet young girl who attended the church. I was further shocked to hear she served as Tina and Scott's housekeeper and cook, as well their constant babysitter. I never completely understood her. She was a young girl, but her eyes were entirely lifeless. I'd heard talk she had gone through quite a bit of pain in her youth and was so confused about her life that she actually ended up living with these two people and their kids. But as far as I could tell, she'd ended up as their *de facto* maid. My heart broke for her. I had to submit to Tina and Scott's craziness once a week; she had to every single day.

Our conversation for this meal was another lap around the exact same track, explaining the start of their church from their mother church in Chicago, but I couldn't stop thinking about Julia.

After the next church service, I went to Tina and Scott and confronted them. "You tell us your prophecies are being fulfilled," I accused. "Where? What are they?

I don't see them. Give me, by name, one good example. You tell me I've been healed, but I'm not. You tell me you are flowing in the spirit, but I see absolutely no evidence of it. I have seen the Spirit move in other people before, people I've grown great respect for, but I'm not seeing that in you. Is this all a show? What are you actually doing?"

Tina was furious she was being confronted. She responded with something I never saw coming. She told me that I was opposed to having a female pastor, that I was not open to her leading the church, which was why I wasn't feeling the movement of the Holy Spirit. I told her that wasn't the case at all. I told her the inadequacies I saw in them had nothing to do with whether she was a man or woman. But what I said didn't matter. God had "revealed to her" that my real issue was with women leading church. She reminded me I grew up in a church that closed off opportunities for women, which was true. Both Amy and I had seen Godly women held back from preaching, but neither of us felt it was right or Godly; we were both forced to follow our parents to church. My issues had nothing to do with her gender, but with Tina's inability to lead a group of people closer to God. Nevertheless, from that moment on, it became Tina's intent to heal me of my chauvinistic ways.

For a while after that, I prayed to enter that place with an open heart to receive new wisdom about what was happening. I *was* even trying to be open to the idea that maybe I was a male chauvinistic pig, but every week I would exit the church even more disappointed. I was tired of allowing these empty spiritual moments, being prayed for, being doused with cooking oil or having my hair washed to rid me of my sins. I said yes to everything until I couldn't take it anymore.

Ryan said his wife, Jenny, was now starting to point out all of his male-oriented views. Ryan and I were baffled. How had this church turned into this crazy gender argument? Ryan finally had enough of it and ordered their entire family, three kids included, to leave the church just before Christmas. Jenny threw a fit, but Ryan, a retired US Navy officer, bravely decided to never let their family show up there again.

Amy went to Chicago with the pastors for New Year's Eve that year. They attended a celebration with the church that had commissioned Tina and Scott, with no previous experience or training, to begin a church in Jenison. This was the same church they would constantly tell us about each week—about how the back room was filled with beautiful, handmade furniture, and how they had gathered around a giant table (at which the pastor sat in his noticeably higher chair) and feasted on the finest meals the city had to offer. These stories made me wonder why the Jenison Church was struggling financially so much. They seemed desperate for money, and I had the thought that maybe Amy was funding the church by donating hefty portions of her photography income.

Early 2011, I stopped going to Regeneration Church, but Amy continued. I was now seen as the lost sheep that had wandered into the wilderness. I knew they prayed for my sinner's soul, that I would "see the light," that I would be "healed from my sins," that I would come to admit my hatred of women, repent, be slain in the spirit, and finally be healed of my cancerous soul.

Ryan and his family stopped going to the church too (initially, against his wife Jenny's wishes). He told me his wife later admitted to having the wool pulled over her eyes. But when they left as a family, she managed to crawl out from under that rock and see how much the church had possessed her. She was extremely grateful to Ryan for pulling their family out of that mess.

It was about this time when Amy instructed me I was no longer to speak with or be around Ryan or Jenny. In fact, she was convinced I was having an affair with Jenny.

I was at my wits' end. I told Amy that if we were to survive this, we needed to move. Anywhere. I was willing to leave my doctors, our friends, our house. Because if we could get out of Grand Rapids, we could start over somewhere new. She was kind enough about hearing this offer but told me she had finally found the place God wanted her to be.

It was intense when I was actually attending the church, but even more bizarre to see Amy coming and going. From this perspective, it seemed that Amy had gone through a complete changeover. She was definitely turning into a different woman, but I honestly didn't know if she was getting better or getting worse. One day, Amy came home from church simply beaming. She knocked on the bathroom door where I was sitting on the toilet. She opened the door with a giant grin on her face and announced that she had bought some presents. "Presents? For who?" I asked. Earlier that day, Tina had prophesied that we would have twins. So, on her way home from church, she purchased two small wall hangings for them. Until that day, our whole decade of being together, she had showed absolutely no interest in ever having children. But now that Tina had prophesied it, it was certain to happen. I was completely dumbfounded. It was that moment, sitting on that toilet, when I realized I was completely surrounded by shit.

Soon Amy began sleeping in a different bed. We shared few words. I had no idea what was presented to her at church because she openly told me she couldn't reveal that to me, but she seemed to accept all of it. When I finally told a few friends about what we were going through, they practically yelled at me: Amy wasn't going to a church, but a cult. I hated the idea of calling it a cult, because my wife was in the middle of it. So, I always reminded them that everyone who went there believed in Jesus just like the rest of our churches, so it shouldn't be called a cult.

But I was starting to wonder.

I get why people are afraid of an active and moving God. I understand that places where God actually shows up can easily get out of hand. There was a reason why people—especially religious people—were over-the-top angry at Jesus while he was on this earth. I get why people pray with unearthly faith that their prayers will be fulfilled. I get why God chooses to move through the obviously weak and not the seemingly strong. I get why people fall to the ground when the Spirit overcomes them. I get why a full field of Ugandans can turn into a cacophony of euphoria after God presents His power of healing. Especially when the only other option we have is to attend a dead church where they sing lifeless hymns as the pastor checks off the boxes of preaching and communion.

But I still can't figure out why in Grand Rapids, a town full of Dutch Reformed Protestants, it was so hard to find a church that was capable of believing in a God who openly and actively responded to His people on a daily basis.

And that was it. That was the reason why Amy and I started to spread further and further apart. Most times, when people ask, I can't bring myself to tell them this story. When I do, they look at me like I'm crazy for sticking around as long as I did. "Why didn't you just pull her out of there?" "Why didn't you just move?" "Why didn't you just tell her what to do?"

The answer was complicated, and this had been the whole issue from the beginning. Amy grew up in a Southern Baptist church and was told by men what to do and how to act for her entire life. She was told what to believe and how to believe it, and then she had a strong woman, Tina, telling her to throw off all those old chains. I totally understood why Amy was so into it. It was her clarion call to become the Christian woman who didn't have to obey the old rules of a woman's role in the church. This was her salvation from her historical family. This was her salvation from her Southern Baptist upbringing. This was her salvation from her father. This was her salvation (apparently) from her husband. This seemed to be her salvation from anyone telling her what to do or what to believe.

When I left the church, disobeying the pastor's orders to stop traveling and speaking, Amy stopped traveling with me. The same message we agreed upon, our joint story to fight cancer with faith in God and alternative treatments until I was completely healed, was now null and void to her. I was traveling, telling of God's past, present, and future glories, while she stayed home, waiting for God's glories to unveil themselves before discussing them. We were on completely separate pages and telling completely different stories.

She dove deeper into her books on prophecy and spiritual issues in the home. She read there were certain animals that were cursed by God and anyone who displayed them was prone to their curses. So, she packed up all the images of owls and frogs from our apartment. She also wanted to get rid of all of our unholy media, so she went through our DVDs and threw 75 percent of the collection into a bag. Then she went through our bookshelf and wiped it clean. Sorry Francis Schaeffer, Rob Bell, and Peter Rollins. Sorry to Khalil Gibran for your foreign sounding name. Sorry Nick Bantock; maybe your magical letters were too sincere, heartfelt, and mysterious to make the cut. Sorry again to my collection of Enneagram books whose cover has a nine-pointed star which, unfortunately, is too close to the six-pointed star of the devil. Good thing I didn't have any Jewish books on the shelf.

She took them all on a thirty-minute drive to Holland where she burned them in her brother's backyard barbecue pit. Jonathan later told me he wanted to steal a few books and movies out of the pile she had put together. Honestly, it wasn't that big of a deal. I had no serious connection to anything she was burning. None of those things were worth any more arguments with her. If she would have simply asked me if she could burn them, I would have agreed. But she never asked me. She just did it.

In August of 2011, Amy and I went to Northern Michigan to go camping. We were still attempting to act married and appreciated the times we were able to do things like this. On the way back home from our weekend trip, the sun was nearly down and the rain was pouring when I mentioned I didn't feel well. At this point, I was still taking pills, performing enemas, sitting in my sauna, and drinking tea to rid my body of toxins. I had decided not to take my enema bucket camping, but I was still taking my pills to regularly flush toxins from my body. And during our trip, I wasn't sweating in my sauna. When we got back to the house, I gulped down two glasses of Essiac tea, releasing even more toxins into my body, before stripping down and heading into my sauna. I hadn't realized how dehydrated I actually was.

Luckily, Amy was concerned enough to sit in the room with me. I sat in the sauna until I became abnormally hot, but on my way out suffered another quick and severe seizure. Amy rushed in to catch my arm to save me from falling flat on the floor. I puked and passed out.

Amy called the ambulance, which took me two blocks down the road to the emergency room where I was admitted to the Intensive Care Unit.

While I was still going in and out of consciousness, Amy had called my younger sister, Heather, and her husband Michael to let them know I was in the ER. They had moved to Grand Rapids about three months before this seizure happened, but Amy told them not to come and visit. They could help best, she said, by going to the house and cleaning up the vomit in the guest room. Wanting to help in any way they could, they did as Amy said before they came to see me.

Apparently, while I was going in and out of consciousness, Amy called Tina and Scott to let them know I was in the hospital. They wanted to come into my room and pray for me. Of course, I have no recollection of this, but I wouldn't allow them to enter my room. Even in my semi-conscious state, I wanted absolutely nothing to do with them. When I came to, Amy chose not to tell me that I refused Tina and Scott's visit, but Heather did. She was familiar with them and aware of the distance they created between Amy and I. So, when she told me that, I recall a sly smile shared between us.

I was back at home by September 11th, 2011, which was the ten-year anniversary of the plane crashes that destroyed the World Trade Center, and the coverage was huge. All day long, NPR replayed news stories and interviewed families whose loved ones had died due to those attacks. They said that, on that day, only three words mattered: The same three words repeated on cell phones from members of the planes to crying families at home; the same three words muttered by firemen running up the stairs nearly certain of their doom; the same three words echoed in homes while watching that historically catastrophic moment. All of us, sharing these same three words: I love you.

Amy and I had originally met in October 2001, and here we are in September 2011. Our anniversary was only one month off from an entire decade of the worst tragedy our nation has ever endured. But in my own personal tragedy, I was mourning the slow loss of my living and breathing wife.

At the end of the day, when the radios were all turned off and the talk shows were over, I knocked on the door to Amy's office. No response. I slowly opened the door and sat down on the corner of her couch like I always did when we would review her final photos or come up with new ideas regarding her business. But this time, she didn't look at me. I wasn't entirely sure I wanted her to. I wanted to say something, not entirely sure how it was going to sound or what response I might get, but I knew it needed to be said. "Amy, if I were on that plane that day, you are the only person I would have called to say, 'I love you.'" And whatever happened next is not enough to stick in my memory or interesting enough to have been recorded in my journal. I imagine what happened next was nothing at all.

TWELVE
PARADISE LUST

I WOKE UP NUMB ON MY THIRTIETH BIRTHDAY, OCTOBER 15TH, 2011.
Significant days like that should be celebrated, steeped in indulgence even. But
that day slowly plodded along. The clock took its own time counting down the
hours until that evening's festivities. I was nervous, considering I hadn't come
up with an answer to *that* question—the question regarding why, on the morning
of my thirtieth birthday, I woke up alone and homeless on my little sister's Ikea
couch. If it's true that life begins at thirty, why do I want to roll over and die?

Heather, who owned said Ikea couch, organized an over-the-top party. She knew
how lonely I felt and had invited friends to join me in the backroom of Bar Divani,
my favorite spot in town. To fully embarrass me, she coordinated with my mom
to put together a slideshow of embarrassing childhood photos (including a three-
year-old version of me in proper British three-piece suits followed by a picture of
me racing around the backyard sporting nothing but my favorite blankie). These
pictures were mixed with collected Twitter-esque comments from party attendees
and dear friends from around the world who couldn't make it that night. Most
"tweets" shared something that made me swoon, while others referenced slightly
inappropriate jokes that made me smirk. I was puzzled at the number of people
who used their limited characters to comment about how I dress. I'd prefer to be

remembered for honor or creativity or bravery, not pocket squares.

Rimple, the bar's general manager and a close friend, had selected exquisite wines and tapas to be served to forty or so of my dearest friends on tables filled with candles. When the time was right, we toasted with our champagne flutes and I blew out the thirty candles sitting on top of the best pumpkin and cream-cheese birthday cake I've ever put in my mouth. The evening was perfect.

Or it would have been perfect without *that* question slinking around the room.

I elected to ignore this conspicuous question by getting drunk. I refused to make eye contact with the giant elephant standing in the middle of my party, the same lumbering beast that followed my inebriated trail back to Heather's couch. Later, when everything returned to quiet, lonely darkness, I lay down, removed my invisible mask, and cried myself to sleep. I still didn't know how to answer *the* question. The same question everyone was kind enough not to ask.

Where is Amy?

For the previous year Amy and I were, in simple terms, failing. Our attempts to understand what each other needed, and what in turn we expected from each other, made us both dizzy. We were on an agonizing merry-go-round. In an attempt to fix this never-ending miscommunication, I suggested a new approach. I asked if we could spend the final two weeks of September away from each other, not talking, but thinking how we could each ease the tension we were both living under. She agreed. It was the longest two weeks of my life. Honestly, I thought we needed a break to cool our heels, that our distance would be replaced by closeness, and that I would return with some type of answer.

But when we met, through what turned out to be yet another mutually misconstrued conversation, Amy decided (or perhaps simply clarified) she wanted to officially separate. In no way did I want this, but she strongly asked me to leave the house. In the confusion of the moment, and to give her the space she seemed to need, I agreed. I knew Heather and Michael would let me stay on their Ikea couch five blocks away.

October was filled with me and Amy's failed interactions, my confused pleading, and, of course, the awkward birthday party. In an effort to give Amy the time and space she was requesting, I eventually found a temporary apartment only two blocks away from her. Michael and I began removing items from our house like a slow-moving funeral procession. Polite neighbors shared quietly pained smiles as they witnessed my ultimate walk of shame. Holding onto the hope of moving back in soon, I chose to leave nearly everything behind. I took only what was essential for living alone for up to six months. Hopefully less, assuming we were able to sort out what had gone so terribly wrong.

I had no issue leaving our house. The issue was with leaving Amy. She had become my home over the past ten years together, the girl I promised myself to forever and ever, "through sickness and health, for richer and poorer." I recalled how Amy was quite explicit in her decision to use the words "till death us do part" in the vows we sobbed to each other in the middle of that West Michigan vineyard. I called Amy "my home" in those vows, with the words I carefully chose to dedicate myself to her. But that October, the worst on record, the only person I wanted more than anyone told me there was little to no hope of us ever sharing a home again.

That November, I rented a newly renovated one-bedroom condo in the aptly named Bachelor Building at 512 Lyon Street. I was told it was originally built for lumber workers in the 1910s. I took a small amount of solace that over one-hundred years ago, a lonely lumberjack sat quietly in the same room. I was alone, which wasn't too difficult. I'd spent plenty of time alone while traveling. The issue at hand now was that I felt alone. My other half, the rest of my existence, sat three hundred yards away. Two simple blocks that felt like a million miles.

I surveyed what I had removed from our house. I had taken one of two beds, one of two nightstands, one of two lamps, one of two living-room chairs, one of two coffee tables, and one of two rockers. My life had immediately become a one-of-two, or maybe a half-of-one—I'm still not sure. I bet lumberjacks never dealt with this shit.

The Bachelor Building contained no colorful mixing bowls. There wasn't a set of kitchen chairs from Amy's childhood we painted black and then sandpapered to proper antique status. There wasn't the office set we purchased to serve as the headquarters for Amy's new photography business. There was no junk drawer, no collections of Riedel wine glasses, and Wüsthof kitchen knives. All of the bedroom furniture was missing. There was no "Trick Dog," Amy's childhood penny-game that somehow filled a similar nostalgic space in my own heart. There were no perfectly rusted-out birdcages filled with old books and piled up hymnal music. There was no one-eyed reindeer Christmas ornament that had been pulled from an attic stuffed with smoke-scented camping gear. There was no design. There was no beauty. There were no memories. The Bachelor Building was recently redone and felt brand-new, but I didn't want new. I wanted my house. I wanted my home. I wanted my Amy.

For the first time in my entire life, I couldn't sleep. I lay awake in bed for hours, sometimes the entire night. My eyes would wander around the empty bedroom, always returning to our familiar grey-striped duvet cover—the same one our cats, Pegasus and Other Kitty, would curl up at the end of. The bed reminded me of how Amy read late into the evenings and how her book light annoyed me as I tried to fall asleep. I would cover my eyes with a folded t-shirt to drown out her late-night hobby. But in my new temporary location, just outside of my bedroom window, was a bright security light shining through the blinds, a permanent reading light. I grabbed a t-shirt, knowing exactly how to handle this new temporary irony.

This was the first time I had ever lived by myself. I had no idea I was so clean. My room was impeccable. I made my bed—the whole bed—each morning. Towels were hung in the same place to dry each day. I cooked, ate, and immediately did the dishes. The toothpaste was squeezed out from the bottom, maximizing efficiency for the next brushing, and was returned to the same place on the shelf. I turned off the lights as I left each room and hung up my clothes each evening. I was a finely tuned machine. But after a month or so at 512 Lyon Street, my finely tuned machine started to feel that same loneliness sinking in. Everything was too organized and proper and dumb.

Yes, living by myself carried a certain straightforward simplicity. I had imagined a perfect life was one where everything was tidy and every task accomplished. But I started to miss the imperfections of existing with another. Maybe true perfection only exists in dealing with another's imperfection. Like when Amy would decide on wearing a stained sweatshirt and ripped-up jeans on Saturday mornings, or when she would shuffle through a messy pile of mail placed on the kitchen table to find the letter she needed, then leave that full pile of mail. Living at 512 Lyon Street, I learned the only thing worse than doing a person's laundry or tidying up after someone is no longer having a person to do laundry for or tidy up after.

It's silly trying to imagine the loss of Amy's impact on me before it was entirely removed. But now, carefully looking back, I see the loss everywhere. I saw the loss of her perfect antique Christmas decorations, which precisely matched my unspoken idea of what a proper Christmas should look like. I saw the loss in coming home to discover fresh groceries in the fridge, while knowing, without looking, where she had hidden her animal cookies. I saw the loss in the scratchy childhood drawings that magically showed up on the side of our fridge, directly from the hands of one of our fourteen nieces and nephews. I saw the loss in her declaration that her cinnamon rolls, the ones she made from scratch, were far too superior to require frosting. I saw the loss when I opened my drawers to find clean laundry, smiling at how my t-shirts were folded in perfect accordance with the DNA-based instructions she inherited from her mother. These brief memories of things she willingly did and their minuscule impact on my daily living may not seem like too much of a loss. But to me, they were.

I wondered if she felt similar phantom pain. I hoped thoughts like "David always used to do this for me" would continually return to sting her heart. She would wake to feed the cats and be pinched at the memory that it had previously been my morning duty. The same thought would cross her mind as she put on her boots late at night, traveling down the spooky back stairs to the dark side of the house to haul our awkward, heavy trash bins to the curb. She'd have to start a new file in her brain for preferred wines instead of trusting my selections on her behalf. She'd have to trust her gut as opposed to calling for an honest second eye on her photography edits. She'd have to calm herself when bats invaded the house from the attic. Maybe she thought of me for a brief moment as she grabbed the cooking pot with the oven mitts and wielded the kitchen broom to begin the catch-and-release process.

As news started to slowly spread of our separation, I found myself saying things like, "I keep praying God will bring us back together." But deep down, I wanted other things. I wanted Amy to be frustrated at her inability to open jars in the kitchen. I wanted her to be struggling in the dark outside our tent, attempting to light campfires with damp wood. I wanted Pegasus to wail for hours, keeping her up when he understood I wasn't coming home. I wanted her gut to feel as hollow as mine did. I wanted to know she was crying herself to sleep, too. I felt selfish for desiring such things, but they were what I wanted.

I would dream of her nearly every night. In my dreams she was always so happy, looking as she did when we first met—young and strikingly beautiful. One night, I dreamt we were driving in our car on the highway and it ran out of gas, just as a massive dark storm was approaching us. I could just make out a gas station on the horizon between us and the storm. I told Amy we still had time to get out and walk to the station before the storm found us. She hesitated, then agreed. We got out and started walking down the middle of the road together. It was cold, so she nuzzled her speckled little pony nose into my shoulder, and I responded by wrapping my skinny arm around her, as though it were considerably bigger and capable of so much more. Then she made a sound, a pleasant sigh, the type of sound a person would make to inform another that everything was going to be okay.

My dreams offered hope for the lonely months ahead, but each morning I would wake in a slight panic and rediscover that reality was quite different. I circled my empty apartment feeling misshapen. The only normalcy I held onto was my daily procedures of enemas, saunas, and pills. This routine became my life preserver, my only constant in these vast, dark, uncharted waters. It became a morning ritual to take my pills, drink a liter of water, make some ganoderma mushroom tea, and brew my special unroasted coffee. Next, I would lie on the floor of my kitchen, usually with a few pillows and a blanket, and perform an enema with the coffee. The caffeine would hit my body like a slap in the face as my fingers twitched through my phone on a search for new NPR programs to listen to. It was normal for me to imagine discussing my story with Terry Gross on *Fresh Air*, or sounding super smart by explaining the intricacies of my brain tumor with Jad and Robert on *Radiolab*.

One morning, lying on my side, I came across an interview with Brook Wilensky-Lanford. She was the author of a new book, *Paradise Lust*, being featured by *On Point* with Tom Ashbrook. The book was a montage of the historical searches for the Garden of Eden, and I was amazed at the illustrative images of these adventurers, these Indiana Jones sound-a-likes from around the world. They spent solid portions of their lives studying Eden folklore, crafting a plan, casting a vision to acquire the funds, and eventually setting sail. Each of them wanted to be remembered in the greatest archaeological find of all time.

The potential location of the Garden of Eden was mapped by the author to include Ethiopia and Mesopotamia. But it listed other options like Northwestern China, The Seychelles, India, Missouri, Ohio, and my favorite—the most mythical of them all—the top of the world. Apparently, a garden buried in North Pole ice wasn't the craziest of ideas, considering that Boston University President Reverend William Fairfield Warren wrote a 400-page book in 1881 proclaiming it as the existence of our Eden. He died holding fast to this belief.

Paradise Lust explained that every culture in history has their own individual story about the "universal myth of a happy garden." This book highlights those fearless thrill-seekers with the guts to venture out to discover that place, as the rest of us sit back and scoff. I found extreme comfort in the idea that all humans at one point shared this single, similar desire. If we go back enough generations, we have a tiny, faded, yet eternal memory of where we came from—a homing beacon still attached to a faint signal calling us back home.

With my eyes closed, mid-enema, I imagined Adam (the guy from the biblical magical garden story) reading *Paradise Lust*. Adam sighed to himself, considering he knew its precise location. He grimaced and made silent corrections to the author's explanations as she hypothesized specific environmental details. Adam would eventually end up crying, something he always did when he imagined what it would be like to return home. I thought how broken his heart must have felt when he was kicked out of the garden with his girl. I pictured Adam waking up in the middle of the night, double-checking to make sure Eve was still asleep, and sneaking out of his side of the bed. He would silently return to the outside of his garden, tiptoeing around the walls, squinting to remember the details of all of the animals he named, and what it really felt like to walk with God in the cool grass. A banishment of such epic proportions—a flaming sword surrounded by angels— would remind Adam of how badly he screwed things up. He would never return home and he knew it.

I felt Adam's heart beating inside my chest. He missed his garden, but I was homesick for something different. I would get up in the middle of a similar black night, sneak out of my side of the bed, and use my permanent reading light to throw on my chunky brown boots. I ventured the million miles to the house that held my home. I closed my eyes as I walked, remembering her honest, wide-mouthed laugh and the lazy gait of her walk. I knew how she would sprawl out in the bathtub to read a book. I knew the exact location of every birthmark, even the one that looked like a dolphin. I knew what she looked like climbing into bed wearing my childhood baseball jersey with "WENZEL" printed in fading yellow letters on the back. These moments were the GPS waypoints for my heart to find its way back home, but like Adam, over time, these images would begin to fade. They'd need much more than my broken memory to survive.

In early December, my frustration reached a breaking point. I wanted to go home. I wanted my relationship back. I started to get serious headaches. I felt my body was nearly out of control. I was warned that increasing levels of emotional stress have the capacity to bring seizures on. I had never actually had a migraine before, but goodness gracious, I finally understood the pain. I couldn't take the painkillers due to my seizures, so I had to wait them out. I was so worn out and this migraine was killing me, so I lay perfectly still in the silence of my bedroom, covering my eyes with my trusty t-shirt. But a looming fear was starting to spread inside me. Headaches are one thing, but serious migraine headaches for a brain cancer patient are quite another.

Nausea set in. I stayed in bed as long as I could before I rushed into my recently modernized bathroom to hang my head over the toilet. The real enemy to any person dealing with seizures is vomiting. The body's natural response to vomiting is the Valsalva maneuver, which increases cranial pressure in the brain cavity. But my brain was too dense with tree branches of tumors and calcium deposits. Throwing up would drastically increase the density, which heightened my potential for massive seizures. I called Heather and Michael, speaking near gibberish, informing them I needed to be rushed to the ER. I hung up the phone and thought, *Okay, help is five minutes away*. Until then, I prayed into the toilet, *Do not throw up*.

I had learned the progressive steps toward a seizure over the past three years. Despite the ongoing car wreck of a migraine between my ears, an entirely random thought entered my head. I had come to discover that the first step of serious seizures is the onset of a single ridiculous idea that made absolutely no sense. That thought would open the door, allowing my brain to slip into an eddy of feverish circular thoughts, not unlike those notions that repetitively haunt us in the middle of sleepless nights. My ridiculous thought was: "Do I edge the yard first? Or do I mow first?" Immediately recognizing this idea as being completely out of place, I attempted to Zen it away from mindful consideration.

Next, the right side of my body started feeling warm and tingly, especially in the joints. Seconds later, I lost all feeling in my right arm. I reached to grab it with my left hand, holding on tightly as though I were keeping it attached. The steps were progressing frighteningly fast. Sounds started swirling around my head as I imagined pulling the cord to start the lawnmower in the backyard of 704 Edgewood Boulevard, my childhood home. The sound of the Toro engine and spiraling blade matched the swirling of my head. *No, stop it. Come back to the bathroom.* My mouth started sweating. *This is not good.* I spat the excess saliva into the toilet. *C'mon, focus!* My taste buds cringed at the taste of heavy metal, a rare memory I recalled from the shower on the morning of my first tonic-clonic seizure. I fought my brain as it visualized my tongue licking the metal blade of the mower, tasting its rusty flavors as they flaked off into my mouth.

Making it this far down the seizure steps rarely happens. I started crying. It had little to do with my physical condition and everything to do with how lonely I felt at that moment. I knew I'd passed the stage of making words, so I started making unintelligible sounds, forcing air up through my larynx. Hearing my voice reminds me I'm still alive. Tunnel vision started settling in over my eyes. I remembered my final thought, but only because of how silly I felt thinking it at the time, "I wish Amy were here." My hands loosened and my body shut down as I crumpled to the floor. In the final half-second before going unconscious, knowing this current struggle would soon be over, I felt incredible peace. I honestly wasn't sure if I would wake up again and, surprisingly, that idea seemed fine with me. I passed out, vomited, and seized on my newly installed black and white tiled bathroom floor.

I woke to hear Heather and Michael breaking into my locked apartment. Minutes later, they had shuffled me into their car and rushed me three blocks to the emergency room.

I was quiet as my body rebooted. I heard fuzzy words like tumor and swelling and surgery as I was wheeled through the back hallways of the ER in what seemed to me like a giant circle.

The pain of my migraine was increasing again as they put me onto an ER bed and switched my hookup to an IV pumping me with potassium and pain killers. It was there, being stretched out onto the hospital bed, with wires and tubes going in every direction, I realized I'd pissed my pants. The brain, even at its lowest functioning capacity, still carries the power to create personal shame. I was embarrassed as these young female nurses took my urine-soaked pants off my wobbly, half-doped up, puke-covered body. I closed my eyes. That meant this wasn't actually happening.

After my quick change, when everyone stepped back into the room, I immediately had another full-on seizure. No warnings this time around. Everyone stood and watched as I convulsed on display. I passed out for who knows how long and returned to find Heather holding my hand. As is typical, I began with the two standard post-seizure questions regarding time and space:

"Where am I?"

"The emergency room."

"How long have I been here?"

"One hour."

"Where is Amy?" I asked. "Was she there when they came to get me?"

Heather paused after hearing that question.

"David, Michael and I came and got you in your apartment."

"I know. Where's Amy? Was she there?"

Heather paused. "We picked you up at *your* place. Do you remember *your* apartment?"

"What do you mean?"

"Michael and I came to your apartment, picked you up, and brought you to the ER."

(Pause.)

Heather backed up further. "Do you remember your apartment?"

"No."

Heather explained the details of my fancy condo in the Bachelor Building at 512 Lyon Street. She covered the shape of the apartment, the kitchen tiles, and antique wood flooring. No recollection. She brought up the remodeled bathroom and the beautifully redesigned, yet leaky, shower. She asked if I remembered mopping up the bathroom floor after each use. Nothing. She dug deeper. "Remember when you moved in, you removed the instructional booklets from the kitchen appliances; the microwave, the oven, the stove, the dishwasher? Do you remember stacking them together and placing them in their own cabinet?" Interesting. Of all things, I remembered that. The appliances had never been used before. Apparently, this was the memory, the mental key that unlocked the door to my new temporary place of living. Details came flooding back to my brain: My rocker, my striped duvet, my green writing desk and, eventually, the harsh reality that I lived there and Amy did not.

This news punished me. I felt I was raised from a deep eternal sleep to be informed I had been left alone. I started to cry, which made Heather cry. She told me that Amy and I had separated and that I had been living alone for more than a month. Not remembering any of the details, I asked Heather a simple question, as though she could answer it, "What happened to us?" Heather rubbed my hand and said nothing. I wiped up my tears and became very quiet for a few seconds. Then I turned back to her and nervously asked again, "Um, where is Amy?" Heather looked at me, perplexed.

I suffered what's called Transient Global Amnesia. I learned what this was by listening to NPR while doing an enema on the floor of my temporary apartment. With this condition, the brain's memory resets every few minutes. My memory was originally two minutes long. Next round it was two and a half minutes, then three. Eventually five. I asked the same questions over and over with the onset of each new memory cycle. The first question I asked at the beginning of every cycle was the same one I repeated lying alone on the couch in the drunken fog of my thirtieth birthday, "Where is Amy?" Heather answered that same question ten times over the next hour, each time hiding her tears. She told me over and over again, "David, you and Amy are no longer together."

Heather had been calling Amy, trying to get her make the two-block trip to the emergency room. At first, Amy didn't feel comfortable showing up. But five hours after my arrival I was relieved to see her walk in. With my recently learned knowledge of our separation, and in the cloud of my morphine-induced haze, I grabbed her hands and told her we would fix it. We'd fix everything, no matter what was wrong. I reached for her face and pulled her lips to mine in the middle of my curtained-off emergency room.

Her lips felt the same as the first time we kissed, nearly a decade earlier, beneath the clock tower in Covington, Kentucky. Later in our marriage, she admitted her hesitancy in returning that first kiss. We'd only known each other a month and were trying to move slowly. But I couldn't help it. I was head over heels in love with her, so I grabbed that lovely face underneath that broken clock tower and I kissed her mouth. In my memory it was the only other time I felt a similar uneasiness behind those lips.

Radiolab taught me about Transient Global Amnesia. They discussed how it profoundly affects a person's memories, allowing their honest unconscious self to be fully present, like taking a dose of truth serum. The patient becomes their "true self" and the memories retrieved point to their deepest core, not too dissimilar from learned behavior or muscle memory. I couldn't explain where I lived or what hospital I was in. I couldn't describe what I did for a living, or recall what year it was. I described the president as "some black dude." I only knew the basic truth that existed deep below everything else: my first name and a strong desire for the presence of my wife. That was all I cared about. Amy was my learned behavior. She was my muscle memory.

The third decade of my life, the one beginning with the worst October on record, I faced the potential end of my marriage. At our wedding, July 23rd, 2005, Amy's and my hands had been loosely tied together with rope. The officiant, Uncle Paul, took a third rope and encircled our hands representing a joint covenant with God in this beautiful Irish tradition. We openly invited God to guide us from that day forward, giving a special nod to our inevitable struggles.

And now, six years in, we (or maybe just I) were aware of how badly things had been screwed up. I would do anything to fix it. I repeatedly asked her for forgiveness and offered it freely to her in return. I wanted us to work, to go back in time, pulling all the shattered fragments from underneath the rug, and carefully begin to reassemble. *Please God, please don't make me the lonely lumberjack.*

I recognized the boldness in those great adventurers who brazenly quested to discover their happy garden, even at the risk of their own public sanity. I felt called to a similar odyssey, to risk essentially everything in my search for home. I didn't care that others told me my garden was a lost cause or even a historical myth. Either way, I knew it wouldn't be found in Ethiopia, Mesopotamia or the outermost regions of Northwestern China. It wouldn't be found in India, The Seychelles, Ohio, or the Show-Me State of Missouri. My paradise wasn't a location at all. It was my blonde girl from Michigan, my flip-flopped bridge-walker, my one-armed stunt woman, my clock-tower kisser. I would do anything to find my way back home to her.

THIRTEEN
HIRAETH

AMY WAS NO LONGER SLEEPING NEXT TO ME IN MY HOSPITAL BED.
Heather and Michael stayed in my room for two of the nights I was there. On my final day there, Heather sent out a text inviting all of my friends to come and join us in the hospital room. She asked if I wanted to invite Amy, but I was positive she wouldn't show up and didn't want to be disappointed by being right. She invited the crew: the Duffys, Ben, Cliff, Seth and Sally, Chuck and Holly. We set up some Christmas lights (a fire hazard, we were reminded) in my room. I was hoping someone would bring some decent grub, but my responsible and rule-abiding friend Cliff went one better and brought beer! So, I had a small sip as everyone else attempted to keep theirs hidden, and we had a wonderful post-seizure, pre-Christmas party in my hospital room. Later, everyone gathered around me and raised their glasses as we toasted to overcoming this cancer.

Because of the seizure, I was unable to drive for six months, until the first week of June. It was a long winter slogging around town in my boots. But my closest friends were aware of this and wanted to comfort me. Amy's brother Jonathan and his wife, Kristen, brought their boys over and offered me a tiny Charlie Brown Christmas tree. Then the Duffys came over and brought me another Christmas tree. It was so special to see these people who cared enough about me to take care of me in these days of struggle.

Growing more and more concerned about the nature of my brain's capacities after my last seizure, I scheduled a meeting with Pine Rest, a local mental health institution, and signed up for a full-day brain test. I went into their office early in the morning and met with a psychologist named Dr. Burkhart. He told me he was going to measure my potential brain activity, then measure those scores against my actual brain activity. He explained we would go through a series of bizarre tests, having me name random items, solve mazes, fit everyday items into a puzzle board while my eyes were covered with a blindfold. I was interested to see if this process and the results would clarify how I was feeling of late. I felt different but wanted a doctor to confirm these changes.

We began. He held up cards with names of colors, like red or yellow, but asked me to say the names of the colors printed in different colored ink, like blue or purple. We did old-school mazes, and I felt I performed okay. But when it came to the puzzle board, placing everyday items into their correct positions while blindfolded, I struggled to match the items in the right holes. Then he showed me photos of simple everyday objects for me to name. I chuckled to myself, knowing this was ridiculously simple: Dog, pencil, computer, candle, and…uhhh.

Looking at this last image, the feeling of panic swept over me. Dr. Burkhart, sensing my pause, asked me, "David, do you know what this is?" *Say it! Tell him what that thing is!* My brain quickly recalled my history with this item. I remembered going into a store in Bratislava, Slovakia, where I purchased this item for myself. I had my granddaddy's sitting on my shelf at home. I had studied this item with Jay for hours and hours on end. *David, come on, what is it?* I must have started sweating in my momentary panic. The doctor said, "Okay, David, it's all right. That's a watch."

Don't you sit there and politely tell me "That's a watch"! I know more about watches than anyone. I know everything about my favorite watch, an International Watch Company Mark XV, which I desperately desired to own one day. I know specific details with all the brands like Chopard, Breitling, Vacheron Constantin, Audemars Piguet, A. Lange & Söhne, Girard-Perregaux, Jaeger-LeCoultre, and Panerai. I even know about Patek Philipe's most famous watch of all time—a watch whose face was designed as an actual representation of the stars seen from the window of its purchaser, Henry Graves. It was easily the most complicated watch ever created, which is why a few years ago it was sold at the highest price of any watch: $24 million.

So, don't sit there and tell me I'm looking at a *watch!*

This strange moment destroyed me, and tears started rolling down my face in front of my doctor. This was possibly the first moment I truly understood how this cancer has affected my brain. To a degree, I *knew* I had brain cancer, but I didn't know *how* this brain cancer had affected me. Medically speaking, my brain was starting to fail, which I knew would eventually occur. But the cursed day had come to prove this failure was already starting to happen.

The doctor came back to me at the end of the day with a confused look on his face. He quietly sat down and paused for a few seconds. "David, we originally tested you for your base IQ, which shouldn't have been affected by this tumor. It showed you are four IQ points below genius, in the Superior Range, with results all landing in the 90 percent and above range. Then we tested you while taking into account your current brain function. We saw weaknesses in the executive function portion of your brain where this tumor is present. Across the board you tested below 10 percent, and in tests like the 'Stroop Color and Word Test' and the 'Trail Making Test,' you scored 3 percent. And one of your tests actually came back at 1 percent. You've lost a large amount of brain capacity in the prefrontal cortex or the executive function portion of your brain, which is extremely important to everyday living. It seems your brain is essentially performing at half the capacity of what it previously was. I'm sorry to have to tell you this."

I had seen images of the mass, heard brain doctors talk through potential medical effects on me, but this was the first time I'd heard the scientifically proven impact of this tumor on my daily life. After hearing and struggling to deal with Dr. Burkhart's words, as I was driven back to my empty, lifeless, barely decorated apartment, I felt myself falling into a deep depression. *Without my brain functioning properly, what would I be? Who would I be? Dear God, I have no idea.*

I told my family I wanted to spend Christmas by myself. I didn't want to entertain or be entertained. I didn't want to be around anyone at all. I just wanted to sit, fully take this news in, and desperately ask God to show up and fix my broken brain.

I became panicked. I had to try something else. Micah had once mentioned another doctor, Dr. Morgan, in Ann Arbor who performed Rife Treatments. Having no idea what that was, I read more about this practice online. In the 1930s, Royal Rife invented a specially designed microscope to view microbes that were too small to view through typical microscopes at that time. Rife invented this device to destroy pathogens by providing frequencies that were the exact opposite of the pathogen's frequency. Essentially, every living being has a wave of energy moving through it, and this machine would send the same frequency of wave, but in an equal and opposite force of the disease. In doing so, the pathogen would quickly die.

Rife claimed that an ongoing conspiracy led to his claims being discredited by independent researchers of the American Medical Association during the 1950s. He claimed he had created the machine to cure the majority of diseases, but the AMA came in and "brainwashed and intimidated" his colleagues. The rumor mill reported that the AMA hired gangsters to destroy his lab by burning it to the ground along with all of his patient documents.

I went over to Dr. Morgan's office, and she ran my first test. Initially, she asked about my overall health, and when I told her I had never been sick, she expected to see that in the results. But after running her first test she found I had near 100 different types of negative pathogens. Of course, she found the cancer, but also found thirteen types of parasites, five types of Lyme disease, Epstein-Barr virus, and so on. She said she was honestly surprised I was capable of walking myself into her patient room.

Christmas wasn't too merry that year.

It was a lonely holiday. On Christmas morning, sitting in my chair, I realized that Amy had left to go visit her family, and I hadn't seen my cats in three months. I walked the two blocks to my house and sneaked inside.

I can't say I've ever seen a happier cat than Pegasus. Other Kitty was excited, but Pegasus was begging for love and attention. I picked him up and, as usual, he was rubbing his head against my ear while his tiny little claws were puncturing my shirt and scratching my shoulders. I took a private tour of our home, seeing how my room had turned into a temporary storage area. Amy's office was filled to the brim with her work, but other than that, everything looked as it did when I left. I sat down in the living room as Pegasus was still pawing all the love he could get out of me.

I checked the closet where we hid our $10,000 worth of silver bars. I was glad to see them still sitting in the back without being moved or sold. I walked to the dining room, where I saw our large wedding picture still hanging on the wall, the image of us proudly walking down the aisle on our way out of the ceremony after just being named man and wife. We're looking at each other with such joy in our faces, ready to take on life together. This. This was all I needed. This was all I wanted.

Before Christmas, Amy had been pestering me with this healing conference coming up soon over in nearby Holland. I didn't want to go because it seemed like another Sunday morning TV special, but I would have loved to go if she came with me. She refused and told me this was something I needed in my life. After much personal debate, I chose to go. I thought this could potentially be something to draw us back together. But who knows? Maybe I would even learn something from it.

It was a two-day conference. Knowing I couldn't ask someone to make that forty-five-minute drive twice a day for my sake, I broke the no-driving rule and drove my car to the conference. I showed up as the crowd slowly shuffled in. I noticed everyone in there seemed both physically and emotionally sick. You could see their maladies as though they were written on their foreheads. They carried their giant Bibles and their recently purchased large notebooks to capture what would be taught. But when the leader of this conference got up there and started speaking, I felt sick again. He was essentially the Brendon Burchard of healing. He had a plan, and if you didn't stick with his plan, you were wrong.

Nevertheless, this gentleman and I believed the same thing: God could heal those who asked for it. We went through the basic issues of admitting our faults to God, asking for forgiveness from Him, as well as making plans to ask forgiveness from others. Then he instructed us to ask for forgiveness about our past childhood struggles that have manifested themselves in bodily issues. Near the end of the day, he went through a list of actual illnesses and the specific sins which typically led to them. Now, this was interesting. Could my brain tumor be related to a specific sin? Maybe this guy did have something I could benefit from. I admit some of the issues with astrocytomas (a Grade III version of my Grade II Oligodendroglioma) could have been applicable to me: bitterness, unforgiveness, insecurity, fear, oppression, and heaviness.

But then the mood changed in the room. His voice started rising about how our iniquities were the sole responsibilities of our sicknesses. And that if we were completely open about our sins, we would never get sick again. He continued, now yelling, explaining the sicknesses our families face, including the death of our newborn infants, are the results of the parents' personal sins. It seemed like his lips began to snarl as he began "preaching," seemingly forgetting the illnesses of some of the greatest Christians in our history, while blaming them for the maladies they experienced. I could not agree with this.

I reported my findings to Amy at Urban Mill, a local coffee shop. I explained a few elements were applicable to me but there were other things I simply couldn't agree with. I asked about her experience at the conference, but she refused to tell me. Then she continued to insist that the reason I had cancer was because I was hiding secret sins. I told her I wasn't. She didn't believe me. It felt like she had some strange agenda about calling me out on my sins instead of fixing our marriage. I missed that grace she originally showed me when I told her about my secret sin. That felt so much more like my Amy, the woman I married six years earlier.

But in that exact same conversation she started crying, actually shedding big lumpy tears, regarding the kids I would have with my next wife. What on earth was she talking about? I was sitting there, attempting to save our own marriage, but in her mind, I'd already gone and married another girl, and she was actually sad about it. You've got to be kidding me.

By the end of that conversation she had hardened herself to the point where she said that since the beginning of our relationship, she had never even loved me. Her only hope she was holding onto was for me to change into the man she wanted me to be. I desperately tried to not believe her.

I left that meeting entirely confused of what to do next. Scott, the pastor of "Degeneration Church," called me up to offer counseling. Despite the overall ridiculousness of having an in-depth and heartfelt conversation with the man who was bamboozling my wife, I took him up on it. After the horrible experience with Amy at Urban Mill, I decided to meet him there, knowing full well I would never step through those doors again. Scott started the conversation about what it's like to have a wife by telling me I didn't "get" marriage. At first, I honestly had no idea what he was talking about. Amy and I had been married for six years, and of course we had our troubles, but I couldn't follow what he meant by "not getting it."

He started by telling me how silly my actions had been to win her back. He started listing them off, like when I dropped off a $50 gift certificate (given to me for my birthday) to Amy for her to eat at our favorite restaurant, The Chop House. He told me that Amy brought it to them and they all sat around laughing because I don't "get marriage." He said if I actually meant it, I should have gone down to the Chop House and gotten a new card and put her name on it instead of crossing out my name and replacing it with hers. I guess I could have done that, but I wasn't even capable of driving at the time. Did they all really sit around and laugh about a $50 gift certificate because I crossed my name out and wrote hers on it?

He also mentioned the flowers. Crap. I knew it. I told him I should have sent more and more often, maybe on a weekly basis. "No," Scott said. "Flowers aren't the issue. Flowers simply wilt and fade. Flowers are meaningless. You needed to give her something more substantive than that." Again, this boggled my mind. *I've been trying everything I can do to talk to this girl and all they can focus on are flowers? Is she not telling them I've been begging, practically chasing her down to talk? Do they think I'm ignoring her?*

Then Scott leaned in. He wanted to get real. He lowered his voice to tell me that about three years before they started the church, he and Tina fought over an issue, and Tina had essentially kicked him out of the house. He was not allowed to come back until he agreed with her argument. To me, that made absolutely no sense. Your wife kicked you out of the house until you "agreed" with her? What about actual conversation? What about loving each other even through miscommunication?

It's easy to see where Amy was picking up on the issue of everything being my fault and not trusting me because I didn't agree with her. Tina had convinced Amy there was no room for actual communication. Now I understood why my options were to agree with Amy or leave the house. And I couldn't even pretend to agree with her, because that would mean I was admitting to having had an affair.

I was so sick of this. I went home and wrote Amy a long letter telling her how much I loved her and begging her to talk with me. In this letter, I remembered and documented all of our special memories and begged her to think of us, both in the past and in the present, as being a team, dedicated to one another and promising we would overcome our future challenges as we pledged to do on our wedding day.

At our house on Crescent Street, we had two lockable doors. We always locked the one at the top of the stairs, but occasionally left the bottom one unlocked when we were home. I wanted to set this letter on the stairs with a few flowers surrounding it, instead of just sliding it through the mail opening. When I arrived, I saw she had locked the bottom door. Not a big deal; I still had keys. But when I went to unlock the bottom door, my key didn't work. She had changed the locks. Welcome to officially being "locked out."

Home. What does that even mean? I started thinking about it, sitting in my bare living room. The concept of home wasn't about a house, but something much deeper. It's about knowing you are welcome. Knowing you are supported. Knowing you are taken care of no matter what happens. It seemed my own home had not only locked me out emotionally but had also now locked me out physically.

As I sat in my quiet apartment over the following days, gnawing on expired saltines and leftover liver pate, I became obsessed with a concept. This white Eames rocking chair I was sitting in was the only "Home" I currently had. I kept working through this idea, applying this foggy concept to each of us. A chair lets us relax, take a break, and not work. Then I thought that maybe this concept could be applied to a nonprofit organization. The idea of buying a simple chair for poor people in need, or a student away from home, to sit in and read, or maybe it could be used by a disabled veteran who felt they had been forgotten.

Each of the recipients would know this chair was purchased specifically for them and represented the people who were praying for them while this chair offered them rest. I even put together a project proposal to pitch to some nonprofit organization, but I knew no one would buy it. It was just my current fascination; representative of my desire to find rest at that moment. What would it be like to sit in a comfy chair given to you by a dear friend with the sole intention of displaying their love and ongoing prayers for you?

What would this look like?

My sister, Heather, had worked for a Thailand-based nonprofit called The SOLD Project and was now working for them long-distance from Grand Rapids. The SOLD Project was dedicated to preventing children from getting into sex slavery by educating them for real, non-exploitive work. Amy and I had signed up to support Heather and Michael, and I was still getting their monthly emails. The next week I received an email from The SOLD Project asking for donations. There were two main things they needed: an air-conditioning unit and a roomful of chairs.

My mind was blown. This education center needed a roomful of chairs so that students could learn how to read, practice new trades, and prepare themselves for a life of making money, *not* prostituting their bodies. Obviously, their idea of a chair was slightly different from the chair I had previously dreamed up, but I felt like God had put this moment directly in front of me.

Knowing this request was specifically for me, I immediately called my sister to tell them I'd buy all the chairs they needed. I had become focused on this concept of somehow giving chairs to the world, when at the same time, the world responded by asking me for chairs. It was another head nod from God. I was *still* not alone.

Knowing God was next to me, I kept trying to chase Amy down. I asked if we could go to a counselor. I told her I would pay and she could pick which counselor we saw. But she refused, saying she would only be counseled by Tina and Scott. I thought I could potentially suffer that madness, but only if I could bring a silent friend. More than anything I needed someone else in the room to actually see what was going on; a person I could talk to afterwards and figure out how to solve this issue. I called and spoke with Tim Stoner, Sonny's uncle, who has become a great friend of mine and is a man I know loves the Lord. He had volunteered to walk this tough road with me, and I thought he would have great insight into the main issue at hand. He agreed to come with me and promised not to say a word. So, I told the pastors I would attend the meeting as long as I could bring a silent friend Tim, with me. They canceled. Their rules or no meeting.

It was getting bad. I asked to meet Amy, and she agreed. We met outside on a near eighty-degree day early in the year. It was strange weather, but not nearly as strange as what was about to happen. We sat down in the middle of a nearby park as she went on about how our relationship would never work. She even mentioned that, one day, we'd come across each other in heaven, offer each other a firm handshake, and move on. I was in shock.

But then she said the word: Divorce. Strangely enough, I had never even considered that as an option. It never crossed my mind a divorce could be the end of all this. She asked what I would do if she went that route.

During these days of living by myself in my temporary apartment, I was continually at a loss for words to explain my situation. I learned other languages have words meaning something extremely specific that the English language simply doesn't have words for. I became obsessed with this concept and began continually searching for them. These are a few of the words that stuck close by me through this time of frustration with Amy.

Schadenfreude, a German word meaning "the pleasure derived from someone else's pain." I figured Amy had to have some sense of pleasure, enjoying watching my agony when I was no longer living at home.

Then there was the feeling I remember having toward Amy in our early days: *forelsket*, a Norwegian word translated into "the euphoria you experience when you are first falling in love."

Or *tatemae* and *honne*, Japanese words describing the motivations for Amy's decisions these past few months, "what you pretend to believe and what you actually believe, respectively."

Then there was *pochemuchka*, a Russian word representing my feelings with God these days, "a person who asks a lot of questions."

Or how about a word to describe me during these days: *waldeinsamkeit,* another German word meaning "the feeling of being alone in the woods."

Also *pena ajena,* a word I feared my friends felt for me given my situation. It's a Spanish word used in Mexico meaning "the embarrassment you feel watching someone else's humiliation."

Then there's *mamihlapinatapai,* a Yaghan word I thought of when Amy visited me in the hospital: "a look between two people that suggests an unspoken or shared desire."

Or *l'esprit de l'escalier,* a French phrase that haunted me after arguments with Amy, literally meaning "staircase wit," or "the act of thinking of a clever comeback when it is far too late to deliver it."

Then there's a Congolese word I knew I should feel but couldn't muster up the strength to: *ilunga,* meaning "a person who is ready to forgive any abuse for the first time, to tolerate it a second time, but never a third time."

But the word that came to my mind in that moment was a Japanese word, *yugen,* a word meaning "to support, stand behind, gracefully allow, yet not endorse." And I told her if she was actually serious about a divorce, I would deny my signature once, saying I completely disagree with it, but on the second attempt, I would agree to sign, saving us both from further court costs of battling it out. After telling her that, my mind went straight toward our cats, "our kids," thinking maybe we could consider splitting them up. I wasn't too concerned about the furniture or our money because I knew all of that could be split evenly.

A few days later, she told me she was positive that she wanted a divorce and had come to grips with the fact that God would approve. When I asked her what "religious" reasoning she has for it, she brought up my affair again. My heart sank. She told me it had happened, but due to the tumor, I had forgotten about it. I asked about when, and she gave a few possible scenarios, but each of them were completely ridiculous. She told me about all the time I spent on the road and how she knew, without a doubt, I had slept with another woman. There was no point arguing with her.

Ilunga.

I was served divorce papers in late April. I took them into the kitchen, but I didn't take the time to read them. They made me sick. As promised, I checked the box to disagree with the divorce and sent them back in.

The level of hurt I felt was unlike anything I'd ever known. I was experiencing complete rejection. I had attempted to work with Amy, but now she was officially, legally, by order of the court, telling me no. I am not sure there is a more hurtful feeling that can be experienced by a human. It's definitely worse than cancer, I can tell you that. It's not a clean death, not *seppuku*, a Japanese term for an honorable death. It's a filthy death, where you see her car around town, where you can recognize her just by an arm in corners of photos, where you watch her walk right by you and pretending she doesn't see you.

After receiving and replying to those divorce papers, I had an interesting dream. Amy and I were outside, and she approached me with me a blue folder. I knew this folder contained the final documents representing our divorce. But when I opened the folder, there were no papers to sign, but a long, orderly row of wood carving tools. Tools to sharpen, to chisel, to dig, or to file down. They were all different sizes and used for different purposes. But they were all brand new. I went to go find Amy and ask her what this gift meant, but she was walking away from me. And no matter how fast I ran, she was still the same distance ahead of me. I could never catch up to her.

Amy had once told me that the color blue in dreams represents the Holy Spirit. And then there were the contents. They weren't divorce papers, but new and untouched woodworking tools. I thought Amy had handed me my divorce papers, but she gave me something so much different, a kit to start chiseling once again.

Later that week, I got a random call from Amy. I was in my temporary, shared office, but the chance to talk to her made me rush outside to avoid being interrupted. She told me that this morning, Pegasus had fallen over and died. My heart shattered. Pegasus, the cat we'd had for nearly our entire marriage, had literally dropped dead. She said he moaned and shook on the floor for about thirty seconds, then passed away.

She asked what I wanted to do. The thought of incinerating his body made me sick. So, I asked if we could bury him at her parents' house an hour and a half away. She agreed. I asked if I could ride with her there, but she said no. So, I called up my sister and her husband, and they left their work to drive me there. On the way there, I wrote my family an email and told them that maybe Pegasus had a little magic left in him. Maybe his death could bring Amy and I to the same broken place at the same broken time, but not because of each other's actions. Together we adopted Pegasus, and together we raised and took care of him. Maybe this equal loss to both of us would allow us to reconnect. Maybe burying Pegasus could be the final moment to save our marriage.

I pulled into the same driveway I had pulled into a full decade ago to see Amy who, at that time, was filled with love for me. But now, Amy greeted me with our dead cat in a pillowcase and signed divorce papers. I determined to be bold, so I went up to Amy and gave her a huge hug. And kindly enough, she returned it.

She carried Pegasus into the backyard as I went over to the barn to grab a shovel. I am pretty sure the last thing we ever agreed upon was the place to bury him. I started digging. Digging through the pain of his loss; digging and thinking through how we could still save our marriage. I would have dug forever if Amy would have stayed by my side. We placed Pegasus in his grave, both of us sobbing as I covered him with dirt. Amy volunteered to shovel more dirt over him for her own grieving purposes. Next, we went and gathered some wildflowers and positioned them in two separate piles over his grave. Then we stood there, not touching each other, but crying over his grave together. And in our mutual heartbroken silence, Amy bent over to fix the positioning of my flowers.

We decided we wanted to say something to him, but Amy, understandably, didn't want to do it together. So, she walked off as I sat there looking at Pegasus's grave. I thanked Pegasus for his life and told him that the best possible thing he could do for us now would be to serve as the moment to bring my wife and I back together. Then I left as Amy came over to say her piece. I went inside to talk to Valerie, my soon-to-be ex-mother-in-law, about the divorce papers while sneaking glances over her shoulder to see Amy standing over Pegasus's grave.

When everything was over, Amy and I met in the driveway, and her rush to get in her car and drive away was a struggle to watch. We had a short, inconsequential, and unmemorable conversation, and they were the last words we ever said to each other.

> *Hiraeth: a Welsh word meaning homesickness for a home to which you cannot return, a home that maybe never was; the nostalgia, the yearning, the grief for the lost places of your past.*

FOURTEEN
THE TENTH LEPER

SHOULD YOU EVER CHECK IN AT ROCK-BOTTOM HOTEL, BE PREPARED. Because at rock bottom, you feel no need to communicate with others. The depression wants you to watch episodes of *Dexter* till three in the morning. The depression convinces you to eat plates of take-out Thai food every night. The depression tells you to drink until you pass out. And all you really want is a good friend to shut up and sit Shiva with you in your deep-sea diving rig at the bottom of your abyss while listening to submerged versions of Radiohead songs.

Still, I needed my routine. My enemas. My saunas. My pills. My body was being detoxed to such a degree that I was actually wasting away due to an undiscovered sodium deficiency, which turned me into a hospital regular. I visited the ER four times in four months. Extreme depression can actually affect your health and, in my case, it increased my seizures. By now I was such an ER regular that at one point, after understanding the natural progression of my seizure symptoms, I drove myself over to the ER, valet parked, tossed my keys to the attendant, walked in, threw my insurance card on the desk, told them I was moments from having a seizure and needed an IV of sodium chloride STAT. I've never seen so many shocked eyes staring back at me.

I finally found a friend to sit Shiva with me in 2012. His name was Ed Dobson. He has a long grey beard, and he's far ahead of me on this lonely road. My friend Ed has lost the initial purpose he had for his life, he's lost his health, including parts of his physical and mental function. Ed Dobson has MLS or Lou Gehrig's disease. He has written several books and is also featured in a series of films called, *Ed's Story.* He was a pastor of Calvary Church here in Grand Rapids, but he chose to retire after receiving his prognosis.

Ed's life has changed a lot since he was the pastor of a right-wing fundamentalist megachurch. It's amazing what a change in circumstances can do to the way you view God. Calvary Church was a massive church where Pat Robertson would come and shake hands as the conservative wing would descend around him in an attempt to win over the red-ish state of Michigan. Ed was their guy, their go-to. He did everything right. Raised his kids right. Presided over the church right. Led an amazing family. He pursued his calling as a pastor with such fervor that when he stepped down due to this illness, he was shocked to see that his phone had stopped ringing. Eventually, he told me he felt as though he was never even a pastor.

From a spiritual perspective, Ed had seen it all. He was embraced by those who embrace, and he was disdained by those who disdain. He was tired, realizing that much of his work as a pastor would one day be turned to dust. Our mutual friend Steve, from a company named Flannel, had introduced us to each other. Lou Gehrig, meet Oligodendroglioma. It's always an awkward introduction, but we were both used to it.

We went to The Sparrows coffee shop and sat just across the room from where I had my first Arcade Fire premonition that something intense was on my horizon. We got some coffee and sat down by the front window. Ed takes his time. On one hand, it's because he has to, but it's also because he sees the world differently from the rest of us. He is no longer in a hurry. He knows that this moment, this coffee, this conversation, is the only thing that matters. There are no congregations to worry about. There are no church fans to corral or promote to. We are two men, each with different stories, and each with different expiration dates.

Neither of us cared for small talk, so I asked the question that had been haunting me. Eager to hear his response, I asked Ed, "Do you still believe you can be miraculously healed?"

This, of course, was a blunt question, posed to a man who knew the scriptures to such a degree that I honestly didn't know what to expect. I felt as if I had just wandered up Mount Everest to ask a dying kung fu master one simple question. I wanted to ask the man who had seen it all, been on top of the pile of success, experienced earthly suffering, and visited the bottom of the ocean, about his specific thoughts on miraculous healing.

I should have known the answer would be quite different from a what I was hoping. Like a good Jewish teacher, he knew better than to quickly respond with a yes or no. Without a doubt he knew I was wringing my hands under the table to hear his response. Ed slowly and shakily took a sip of his espresso, using two hands to make use of his remaining working fingers to hold the cup steady. His voice is high and crackly, and you can barely see his mouth moving from behind his giant beard.

"Well, David, that depends. Do you want to be healed or do you want to be cured?"

I had never really thought about the difference. I smiled, knowing his Jewish strategy was to ask me a good question in response to my question. "Umm, both I guess," my best German response requesting the most efficient answers in return. I sat quietly and asked, "Is there a difference?"

Ed paused, smiled, looked back at me and suggested a story. He told me of what Jesus did in Luke 17:11-19. The story goes…

> It happened that as he made his way toward Jerusalem, he crossed over the border between Samaria and Galilee. As he entered a village, ten men, all lepers, met him. They kept their distance but raised their voices, calling out, "Jesus, Master, have mercy on us!"
>
> Taking a good look at them, he said, "Go, show yourselves to the priests." They went, and while still on their way, became clean. One of them, when he realized that he was healed, turned around and came back, shouting his gratitude, glorifying God. He kneeled at Jesus' feet, so grateful. He couldn't thank him enough—and he was a Samaritan.
>
> Jesus said, "Were not ten healed? Where are the nine? Can none be found to come back and give glory to God except this outsider?" Then he said to him, "Get up. On your way. Your faith has healed and saved you."

I realized Ed was showing me there were two separate things happening in this story. He explained that Jesus sees a difference between curing and healing. Jesus can cure anything. In fact, in this story he goes on to cure ten people who, as far as we can tell, had very little faith outside of, "Jesus, Master, have mercy on us." Yet one, almost as if he had mentally put the pieces together while walking, turned around, and returned to give thanks and glory to God. This man was cured with the others, but Jesus then says, that since his response to the curing was giving glory to God, his *faith* was the source of his healing. The others were cured. But this man, in addition to being cured, was healed. He had found peace with God.

Ed continued, "Through conversations over the past few years, it seems most people, mainly Christians, like to define healing as the opposite of being sick. But the opposite of being sick is having a cure. We've all visited the doctor when we were sick who says, 'Take this prescription, it will cure what ails you.' This is merely a physical issue, whether God is involved or not." Ed paused his small, slow voice as he used his two shaky hands to take another sip. "I know many people who have been cured but have not been healed. And I also know many people who have been healed but have not been cured."

I started to catch onto what he was saying. The primary desire of a sick person is to be physically cured, much like the nine men cured of leprosy. The primary desire of a spiritual person, or a person aware of their sin, is to be healed, like the tenth leper. The difference between the two words was starting to define itself in my mind. Maybe I'd been barking up the wrong tree, feeling continually let down by a God who "promised" me healing, when in all reality, I had little idea of what healing actually meant.

I believe I will die one day. I believe I will go to Heaven and will no longer have cancer. I believe that my spirit and my soul, regardless of my body, has already been cured of this disease. Cancer may or may not take my life, but I already believe I have beaten death. Cancer has been defeated in my future. I am eternally cured of cancer because I believe that Jesus Christ is who he says he is. So, the question is, why am I so concerned about being "cured" right now?

I realized that over the past few years I had wanted my life to be a beacon, a lighthouse, a city on a hill, and in order to do that I needed to be cured—physically rid of cancer—to show that God is who He says He is. However, I was using the word "healing" as a remedy for the physical disease of cancer. But it's not the right word. Ed was pointing at something entirely different. Healing, the way Jesus referred to it, was about my relationship with God. It also included the relationship I have with myself, with others in my life, and with the circumstances in the world around me. But I realized that, in 2012, the most important relationship in my life was broken.

I was trying to figure out who God had become to me. I was still full of shame and guilt about how my relationship with Amy had turned out. I was struggling to figure out how to "beat cancer," to pray the right prayer, to go to the right workshops to learn how to be cured. But there is no point focusing on curing cancer, a disease I now believe I have eternally defeated, when I truly should be determined to find healing in this life here on earth.

I believe that conventional medicine, alternative treatments, diets, exercise, mystical pendants, healing oils, and Vitamin C supplements all have the capacity to "cure" you, with varying degrees of effectiveness. In fact, I truly believe the human body has the capacity to cure itself on nearly any physical level. But Ed was referring to healing as something entirely different. He is referring to true healing as peace with God, through Jesus. That is true shalom.

Ed told me that those who believe in the peace of Jesus Christ believe they have already been *eternally* cured, no matter what illness befalls them. They believe the sicknesses of this world will be left behind when we reach heaven. So, it really doesn't matter what you die from, be it MLS, cancer, or a plane falling from the sky. Yes, we all die, but by believing we are eternally cured from all sickness, from all disease, from all sin, we no longer are afraid of death. In fact, we sing, "Death! Where is your victory? Where is your sting?" There is none. Jesus has already taken care of our death penalty. So why are we so afraid of illness and death?

"However, while on this earth," Ed explained, "it seems like very few people care to pursue true healing. People go to church, worship a God they barely know, then return home to their broken understanding of how God views them. They sing praises to God while worrying about their social media. They declare their love for Jesus while ignoring their neighbor. They worry about every aspect of their life while never actually believing that God has promised to offer them peace in all of their circumstances."

True healing is "True Shalom." True shalom is what allowed Stephen in the New Testament to forgive those who stoned him. True shalom is what allowed the three being thrown into the fiery furnace to say, "But if we aren't saved..." True Shalom was the fuel for Paul as he struggled through his life.

"True Shalom," Ed said, "is our greatest goal. Death just happens to be a minor detail in each of our eternal stories. Not being sick isn't much of a long-term goal. It's a physically oriented circumstance, driven by fear, with the capacity to keep you from finding shalom. However, by dealing directly with the cause, by finding internal peace with God, it's amazing what the physical body can do. When you deal with the original cause of the disease, be it physical, mental, emotional, or spiritual, the physical symptoms seem to fade away."

I had been practicing this through alternative medicine, using enemas and the Rife machine to get rid of the junk in my body that was allowing the cancer to continue living. I was so focused on the actual symptoms that I'd lost track of what the true, root causes were on the spiritual level. A cure is what a doctor can offer. True shalom—healing—is what God offers. There comes a point when you realize that it is only God who not only eternally heals but also has the power to cure at the precise moment when it will be fully returned for His glory. That may be right now or ten years from now. Only He knows. But it also means that He may or may not offer this cure while you are alive on this planet, but it definitely, without a shadow of a doubt, includes the promise of an eternal cure upon your entrance to heaven.

Ed tells me to pursue peace with God above all else. He tells me to pursue peace and love with myself and with others. He tells me to pursue peace by getting rid of my fear in all of my circumstances. I'm not sure I ever was afraid of cancer. Maybe in small moments when I was in pain, or in moments of high anxiety, doubled over the toilet before vomiting or entering a seizure. But I don't think I have ever been afraid of the oligodendroglioma, the actual tumor inside my head.

But I am scared of God. I often doubt whether or not God can love me. I'm scared of the deep recesses inside myself, the places I don't want to face, fearful of what I might find. I'm intimidated by others and the power they seem to have over me. I am terrified of Amy. I am certain I am not seeking shalom. I am just looking for a quick fix. I just want to tell everyone that God showed up, healed me, and now everything's cool again. What I didn't know is that I needed deep-seeded spiritual healing.

To be brutally honest, I understand why God has not healed me yet. He knows I'm not ready for it. If I were miraculously "cured," I would have so quickly forgotten about these moments when my heart was so open to God. I'm glad I wasn't healed on stage in Uganda, where no one I knew would be a part of it. I'm glad I wasn't cured by Tina, crazily yelling at me just before trying to push me over. I'm glad the end of my story isn't being cured by the hands pressed all over my body as I'm sitting in the middle of a dog pile. I'm glad I wasn't cured in a weekend healing session lead by a skeezy televangelist. Now I can see there has never been any peace in those situations.

God knows the timeframe for me to heal, to be transformed, and to find true shalom. And I should know that during this time, I would make a variety of mistakes, choose wrong treatment plans, believe horrible theology, and numb myself to near non-existence. But God has yet to give up on me.

Ed helped me realize I wanted healing much more than I wanted curing. I realized I've already got cancer licked in the long term. But I wanted healing right now— in my relationships, in my family, between God and myself. I wanted peace with Amy. I wanted to live my life with no fear despite the ridiculous scenarios I find myself in. This will feel like living, despite whatever cancer does to me. Now that I have chosen to pursue healing, I realize the choice of if or when I will be physically cured is no longer up to me.

Having understood the difference between the terms "healed" and "cured," I asked Ed again, "So, as you pursue your eternal healing, do you also ask for an earthly cure from God? Have you given up or do you still pray for a cure?"

Ed raised his eyebrows, not showing focused determination or a desire to control his Maker. His response rolled off his tongue as though he had said it a million times before. He repeated the prayer of Blind Bartimaeus, who, I imagine probably looked and sounded a lot like Ed with his shaking hands and raspy voice, *"Jesus, Son of David, have mercy on me."*

I wanted easy answers. I wanted a cure right away. I hated waiting, so I had wanted it to happen and, if possible, look fancy so I could get paid to keep talking about it. I've learned there are all sorts of tricks you can use if you ever do get sick. You can play worship music all the time. You can repeat prayers of healing to yourself or download a track of healing verses and put it on repeat throughout the night. You can buy bottled water from around the world that's been proven to heal. You can always have your healing napkin on you, not unlike the one I just received in the mail that was apparently blessed by someone important. You can have the elders lay hands on you, or you can step up onto a stage and, before a crowd of rowdy witnesses, have a spiritual breakthrough, fall over, and start shaking. But I'm starting to think that when a person is pursuing healing through seeking True Shalom, the only prayer they need to repeat is, *"Jesus, Son of David, have mercy on me."*

FIFTEEN
LEAVING IT ALL BEHIND

I WANTED TO RUN AWAY from my oncoming car wreck of a divorce, so I made a plan to get out of town. Unfortunately, I was completely out of cash. I had previously invested $1,000 into KIVA, a phenomenal organization providing microloans for those people in developing countries with great ideas but no money to bring them to life. Withdrawing that money from the program made me feel like I was stealing from the poor.

Then I went down to Merrill Lynch and cashed in my retirement account for a few more dollars. I used the points on my debit card to scrape together a little more money. Next, I sold my 2000 Volkswagen Jetta. The car was paid off and worked incredibly well, but I needed the cash. My Skymiles account was massive, and I was ready to burn through all my miles. I had stayed my six months in the apartment, and it was time for me to leave. I packed a single large bag, stored the rest of my furniture and clothes in the shared basement storage of the Bachelor Building, and headed to the airport. The next part of my life after signing my divorce papers would begin with a wedding.

I flew to Los Angeles to meet up with my boys, Santino Stoner, Corey Petrick, Jason Murray, Josh Salmons, and Carl Helder. We all drove up to Santa Barbara to attend Sonny's wedding ceremony to Francesca Giamo, a makeup artist from Los Angeles. Someone had the idea to buy dollar coins so that we could place bets with each other all weekend. It was fantastic. We played cards, went skeet shooting on top of a mountain in Santa Barbara, bet on absolutely everything, and played some random dice game that took up all our down time.

We had the wedding and the reception in the backyard of Fran's father's incredible house. Her dad had made his money in advertising (the creator of *Mad Men* actually visited him to inquire about all of the details of marketing back in the day), and his gorgeous house was filled with amazing Italian food and Italian wine, but the company was so much better.

When the wedding was over, and we'd had a little bit to drink, Francesca's dad let me hop into the driver's seat of his 1958 Alfa Romeo Giulietta. I told him I hadn't driven in six months due to a seizure, but when he saw how happy I was gripping the Italian leather wheel, he told me to move over to the passenger seat and took me on a wild ride around Santa Barbara. It felt like heaven as we drove around that beautiful, hilly beach town, with a revved-up engine in that convertible masterpiece.

The day after the wedding, I drove down for dinner with Jasmine and J.D. in Irvine. They took me to an incredible Mexican restaurant. Again, I tried to outsmart J.D. on purchasing the meal. I promised I'd spend my last remaining dollar on this dinner as a way to say thank you for their help through this situation. But he was too smart for me. Apparently, he gave them his credit card before we even sat down. I stayed at their place that night, sharing stories, hesitantly asking if they knew what was happening with Amy, but they didn't have any answers for me. I think they knew, but I respect them for not letting me know. Jasmine and J.D. were terrific and supportive friends to both of us throughout all of this.

After my days in California, I flew into Omaha. Unfortunately, my computer crapped out on me during the flight. But sure enough Tim Spiker, a client and great friend of mine who knew what I was going through, offered to buy me a new computer on the spot. After surviving that scare, I spent my nights dancing at Jay and Brent's new club, House Of Loom. They brought in a karaoke machine, gave me all the free drinks I wanted, and took me to an after party where everyone ended up stripping down and cannonballing into the pool.

This resulted in an early morning hangover-induced breakfast at Perkins, where we told them to make us the biggest omelet possible. They showed up with a massive pan holding an omelet made of one hundred eggs. We had switched to coffee by this point, but we ate everything in sight. I went home for a two-hour nap before I had to meet up with my dad to celebrate Father's Day at a College World Series game. Jay showed up with his dad, and as we sat in the blazing sun, we bemoaned our activities the night before.

After the game, the four of us went over to Happy Bar, an old dusty bar a few blocks from the stadium. When we sat down to share a beer, it struck me. I had never been in a bar with my dad and shared a beer across the table with him.

It seemed like a moment we desperately needed but never had the guts to pursue out of fear from what would happen. What happens when a father and son have enough alcohol to finally loosen up and speak honestly with each other, as opposed to hiding behind these false religious projections of themselves? But then again, I admit my dad gave up drinking because while we were living in England, I was the three-year-old kid who sucked down two glasses of red wine when no one was looking and got seriously drunk. I was passing out in my high-chair as my mother was attempting to sober me up by feeding me. But from that point forward, I had never seen my dad take another sip of alcohol until the day before my wedding. But even if it was for the first time, I was glad to share a beer with him that day.

I returned to Grand Rapids for a few days and made a few late-night trips out to Oval Beach. I also watched some great shows by Andrew Bird, Brandi Carlile, fun, Sleigh Bells, The Beach Boys, and Garrison Keillor's "Prairie Home Companion," after which Garrison popped my jean-jacket collar as we discussed the benefits of denim versus seersucker.

After that I flew to Portland, where I stayed at Jason Murray's apartment. It was summer, and Portland was in full swing, so we went to the Northwest Music Festival to see Sigur Ros, Beirut, and the Tallest Man on Earth. Jason was being scouted as a designer by Nike, so we visited their incredible headquarters (which was more like a sports museum) in Beaverton, an hour outside of Portland. Jason and I took the train up to Seattle, where I saw one of my best friends, Jon Brown, and we swirled around the beaches, restaurants, and bars before taking the train back home to Portland.

My summer was moving forward in this temporary personal vacation in order to forget what was actually going on in my life. Those months were incredible. Something new every day, new people, new food, new cities. I absolutely loved it. But deep down, I knew I was only enjoying it because it took me away from my reality.

I had to go home because Amy and her lawyer had set up a mediation meeting to determine who got what. I had little to no money to hire a lawyer, so Ryan Duffy (who had just graduated law school) was kind enough to offer his legal services pro bono. When I arrived, I learned Amy had requested two separate conference rooms for this conversation to take place. This felt like such a punch to my gut. She didn't even want to be in the same room as me. Each of us sat and talked with the mediation layer, then he would disappear for twenty minutes to talk to the other party.

The lawyer came in and essentially asked what I needed to survive. I responded with what I thought was obvious: an even split with savings, debt, silver bars, and furniture. But my response seemed like a complete surprise to him. I told him to go tell Amy this should be quite simple: I just wanted half of everything.

He came back saying that due to her higher income, she had actually purchased the majority of the items in the house, including the silver, so they weren't on the table for discussion. I was in deep shock. Ryan and I quickly realized this conversation was going absolutely nowhere and said that we had to do some more thinking about how to handle this situation.

When he left to relay that message, I started wandering around his office, mulling how this meeting even came to be. I tried to figure out why Amy thought she had paid for the majority of our possessions? We were both making good money in those years and each of us could have easily survived on our own. I hadn't kept track of who had paid for what—I just assumed it all belonged to both of us. Ryan was in shock as well, going on and on about how bizarre this entire scenario was. When I wandered over to this lawyer's credenza, I noticed a framed photo of his family. It featured him, his wife, and his three beautiful blonde daughters all in their twenties. Amy's lawyer knew exactly which mediator we needed to meet with. The man with three daughters who all looked exactly like Amy. I just got played.

When I got home I noticed the letters from her law firm preparing me for upcoming legal actions needed. Every single piece of paper read "DAWN: Divorce Attorneys for Women." According to their website, they serve women who needed protection, women who need someone to stand up on their behalf, who have been harmed, who needed fair treatment. I can only imagine what she told them about me. (Years later I was told her lawyer, Megan Lipford, was being sued for legal malpractice in divorce situations similar to ours.)

Amy and I continued to email back and forth about the worth of the furniture.

She created Excel spreadsheets detailing the original cost, current cost, value, the worth of our silver, and the worth of our savings. It got so convoluted, I told her I had to think all this through. I was getting the itch to drop everything. Maybe I should just give her absolutely everything we owned and stop all of this painful arguing. I remembered hearing these words from Ed Dobson's mouth: "If I wanted peace, I needed to be willing to give up everything to obtain it."

Frustrated, I traveled back out to Portland. I was beat. My fourth month on the road while living out of a single bag. I went to stay at Don's new place by the river for three weeks. Portland's transportation system is incredible, so I would take their city train into town and hike all around the city. But this time everything felt different. It wasn't as sunny. There was a little more rain. It seemed the city was slowing down to match my own sadness.

Don told me he was going on a speaking tour, so I had the house to myself for two weeks. He was so kind to me. He told me I could eat anything I want, showed me how the TV worked, how the music system worked, how to access the garage ("so feel free to take my car wherever you need to go"). I was reminded again about what it means to have great friends who come around to support you in times of need.

I had been scrounging around Don's kitchen eating anything I could find but knew I needed to get out and do something. I called a few people to ask what I should do and the majority of them came back with the answer of Mulholland Falls, a beautiful waterfall located about an hour away. I was broke beyond broke and wasn't supposed to get paid for a recent project for a few more days, but I got into his car and pulled out onto the road. As I was driving off, I saw Don's fuel gauge was low, and I had absolutely no money to fill it up. Hoping the gas tank was fuller than it said, I took off.

I made it to the falls and spent the day hiking around. I walked around eavesdropping on the conversations of families, young lovers, and grandparents. I so badly wanted Amy to forget all of this divorce talk. I wanted her here with me, with her hand in mine as we walked across the bridge, coming up with crazy ideas about who or what would survive a fall from the top, wondering about where all this water came from, all the while discussing where we should eat on the way back. That was my Amy. This was her spot. I wanted her to be there with me, not typing up another list of items we owned. I drove back to the house on fumes and wrote Don an apology letter for clearing out his cabinets and his gas tank.

I returned to Grand Rapids, where Amy and I ended up in the middle of yet another email battle over our possessions. I was still staying at Heather's home, sleeping on her couch, when one night, while eating chili by myself, another partial seizure came on. Typical. I stopped eating and waited for it to pass. Then, out of nowhere, my head started jerking to the right. This had never happened before! My neck muscles were out of control, the movement growing and growing till my head was jerking as far as it could. I couldn't stop it.

I ran into the bathroom to look at myself in the mirror. Was I going to pass out? No, I wasn't feeling weak, but I just stared at myself in the mirror as the muscles in my neck took over my head. Again and again, my head whipped itself to the right for over an entire minute. The right side of face went numb, my mouth started to contort and the chili started falling out of my mouth on to the floor. I had no idea what this was, but it deeply scared me.

I had to escape again. I decided to go down to Columbus, Ohio to attend a football game with my dear friend Seth Martin: Nebraska versus Ohio State. After selling my car, I asked my buddy, Chuck, if I could drive his Toyota Yaris. As I drove toward Ohio, the temperature started dropping and rain started coming down. I was on Highway 75 nearing the Pioneer Sugar tower close to Flag City, Ohio when I saw a mobile home seventy-five yards in front of me pop straight up. It had hit another car. Due to the inclement weather everyone was traveling about 50 miles an hour, so it frightened me when the cars in front of me all started swerving, hitting each other, spinning around and stopping, each ending up pointing in different directions. But I had seen this accident in plenty of time and came to a stop about twenty yards before all of the wreckage started.

But then I heard the deep screeching of tires behind me, so I looked up at my rearview mirror to see an eighteen-wheeler jack-knife and spread across all three lanes, its momentum carrying it directly toward me. Realizing it was going to pound into the back of my car, I put the pedal to the metal. As I sped up, I looked back at the rearview mirror to see the semi was still gaining ground on me. I veered to the left of the accident in front of me before I saw the semi-truck slowing down to a stop. Luckily, I was the only car between the accident and the truck. The long truck had nearly flipped onto its side and had stopped in the middle of the road, perpendicular to the highway, blocking all traffic from going around it.

I jumped out of my car to see passengers slowly getting out of theirs. I started yelling at the others to turn off their engines. It was about a six-car pileup. All of the other cars had damage to them. I looked to see a car, facing the opposite way, a few feet from where the semi had stopped. I ran over and looked inside. There were two college girls in shorts and tank tops who were in shock. I took off my hoodie and wrapped it around the girl in the driver's seat and told them to close the door and stay there while I went to check on the other drivers.

I met the others involved in the accident as everyone tried to calm down. The guys with the mobile home actually had a video camera on and were obsessed with trying to figure out how to rewind the footage to playback the accident again. I looked around and realized I was the only car of six that didn't get hit or spin out of control. Plus, I had just dodged death with that truck coming straight for Chuck's miniature Toyota Yaris. Based on what I saw in my rearview, that semi-trailer probably would have taken my head off.

In the middle of giving my report to the police, I turned around to see those young girls being laid onto stretchers and loaded into the back of an ambulance, one of them still wearing my favorite $300 Thom Browne sweatshirt. The sirens wailed and they took off. I honestly fought the urge to yell at one of the cops to call in and stop that ambulance in order to save my sweatshirt. Finally, the police officers told me I could leave. The wreckage in front of me didn't take up the entire road. I felt I could squeeze through, but the officer told me to take an exit that was accessible from where we were. As I exited underneath the same highway I was on, I looked in the opposite direction to see the headlights of stopped traffic all the way to the horizon. I was the very last car in front of the semi, so I pressed on with no other cars on the road.

As I was driving, my brain shut off. I was continually replaying that oncoming semi in the back of my head. I don't know if it would have injured me or even killed me, but it was an incredibly intense moment. When I returned to consciousness, I realized I was the only car on the road. Nothing ahead or behind me for as far as I could see. The semi-truck had blocked all traffic on this exit which was fed by the highway. I looked down to see I had been cruising at about thirty-five miles an hour while my mind took a brief holiday. And for some strange reason, I stopped the car and sat still in the left lane of the highway. I thought back and felt the pain of losing that sweatshirt, the one I loved so much. But then realized, I was still alive. *I am still alive.* That sweatshirt was just a thing, but all those lives, those relationships, those kids, those dreams had just been put into danger. At that moment, for whatever reason, I was still concerned about my overpriced sweatshirt? Wake up, David!

On that empty highway, sitting completely still, it hit me. When that hoodie sped off under blinking lights, I lost something I loved, but I was still alive. If I can do that, why can't I let go of everything I have? I felt that my life and Amy's were quickly approaching imminent danger of being mangled under an approaching semi, but there was I, concerned about my pricey sweatshirt. I decided then and there, as I accelerated to cruising speed once again, to forget the sweatshirt. To forget everything. Amy could have it all. She won, but unfortunately, Nebraska lost to Ohio State 63-38.

I told my family I was tired of fighting and had decided to give Amy everything. Everyone argued, saying I couldn't do that. They told me I worked too hard to own that stuff. And what would I do with no furniture? Ugh, my furniture. I had fallen in love with our furniture. Everything was walnut, the Eames dining chairs that lined our classy, long and lean walnut dining table, next to the walnut dining room buffet. In the living room we had two Eames rockers, two lovely walnut coffee tables, next to our lovely slim blue couch. The kitchen was filled with expensive wine glasses and cooking materials. We had a beautiful home, and we filled it with beautiful things. But after being chased down by a car-crushing semi, I was reminded that I am still alive.

Still unsure about this bizarre decision regarding our possessions, I called Bob Goff. I had spoken with him before, so he knew what was going on between me and Amy. I asked if, legally, it was okay for me to give her everything. Would this in some weird way come back to bite me in the future? Bob's voice raised, as it does, "No! It wouldn't! That'd be such a great caper!"

"Caper" is a word Bob defines as a prank that will be eternally celebrated. He got excited as he agreed with my idea, telling me to show her love with everything I had left, but sure, give everything else back to her. I let out a sigh of relief. Good, I may be crazy, but I'm not the only crazy one. Then Bob asked how long we were married. I told him nearly seven years. He gave me an idea for my next caper, telling me I should go buy seven flowering plants and in the middle of the night, plant them in her front yard for each year of our marriage. I had to laugh. Bob was always going over the top with everything. I told him we rented that house and our landlord already had a plan for our garden and I didn't want to mess it up. But Bob told me he was proud of me and he'd do anything to support me through this process.

When I got home, I wrote Amy an email. It was short. I told her she could keep everything. If she agreed, I would return what I had taken and pick up my storage in the attic along with the rest of my clothes. Rather quickly, she wrote back and agreed.

After Amy agreed to keep all of our furniture, all of our joint savings account, all of our silver bars (now currently worth $20,000), and I agreed to pay back my half of our debt, the details were finished. Unfortunately, she chose to keep my name. She didn't want to abandon the name she'd found so much photography success with. Amy had received what she wanted, and I no longer had to plead or argue with her. We were both pleased with that ending. And with that being settled, the final divorce papers were signed and sent in.

My mom came into town, most likely because she was concerned I'd throw myself in front of a train. I asked her if she would help me take back everything to Amy's. I set up a time with Amy through email, and after loading "her" things onto a truck, I took it back to Crescent Street. I walked in to see Other Kitty, but sadly no Pegasus. I turned the corner expecting to see Amy, but it was some random girl, unknown to me, lying on our blue couch. Amy hadn't even stuck around to say goodbye.

I saw Amy had packed up boxes of my childhood photography books, old cards from friends, and things from my childhood. Must have taken her quite a while. I wonder what she was thinking of while doing that. I wondered if she was sad or happy; sad about the loss of her marriage or happy about getting me and my things as far away from her as possible. I let my mother, who suffers from a weak back, sit out as I struggled to return the furniture. I returned our one of two nightstands, one of two lamps, one of two living room chairs, one of two coffee tables, and one of two rockers. Oh, those beautiful rockers. I'm sure if I'd asked, she probably would have parted with a rocker, but again, I just wanted this to be clean. *One day, I thought, when I am making money again, I'll buy another rocker.*

I saw that Amy had dutifully lined up pieces of paper with instructions on where to sign my name in order to give back the small portion of her photography company that was under my name.

Then I noticed the empty space above the living room buffet table. The wedding picture of Amy and me had been taken down. And that was it. That was when I knew our marriage was officially over. It wasn't the confusion with our mediator. It wasn't the court signing off on an official raised stamp document. It wasn't the disagreement of who gets what. It was when this giant, beautiful black-and-white photo of Amy and me walking down the aisle at our wedding ceremony, with smiles on our faces and shared dreams for our futures, was taken down. That was the end.

I wanted to write down all the reasons why we are so good for each other, and I wanted to give them to her as proof. Proof that we weren't a waste. Proof that we knew, if just for a single moment, we really had found true love. But these words were all stuck in my mind. So instead of giving up with feeble paragraphs, I simply wrote, "There is not a moment I regret. You have been, you are and will always be, loved by me."

I walked out with everything I had before I met Amy, which wasn't much. But I walked out feeling good about myself, about the peace I had found in this relationship throughout these bizarre circumstances. And strangely enough, I felt peace about my relationship with my God. Amy and I were two people, each with information we believed to be God's honest truth. Truths that each of us used to either help or hurt each other. I hope that in any relationship, two human beings who have dedicated themselves to each other could learn to take a giant step backward and remember the big picture. I am as guilty as anyone else when it comes to this, but in the end, we let our religion ruin our love. And as I walked away from what was now her apartment, I pulled out my phone and deleted all of her contact information and slipped my wedding ring into my pocket. My marriage was over.

SIXTEEN
ON BEING ORDINARY

I REALIZED HOW STUPID I FELT when Lori Slager, the owner of The Sparrows coffee shop, wrote me an email to set up a time to meet. I had been going to her coffee shop for over six years, yet never asked what her name was. I had never even introduced myself. It's that type of awkwardness where you feel miserable, but you also feel miserable for the other person because you know they are standing in the same shoes. When I came in, she and I sat in the front window facing the street as she told me about her new nonprofit business she was looking to grow. It was called the Creative Youth Center. She meets with local at-risk kids and holds classes with them after school to protect them from the dangers in their neighborhoods. She told me horrific stories of kids being beaten, forgotten, and raising their younger siblings, and how many of them have no ability to do anything with their future but carry on within this cycle of abuse. Her goal was to end this problem in Grand Rapids. I added them as a pro-bono client for RobinHood Ink. and volunteered to work with them to fully develop this new brand.

I had been taking so much from the world around me, searching for anything I could find to make me feel normal, so the idea of giving back felt wonderful. We had several meetings before we determined the center should be named Captain

H. Tanny's Adventure Trade and Supply Store. The basic premise would be that Captain H. Tanny is always on the road, sending postcards back to the kids. And whenever we had an event, Captain Tanny would write back at the last second. We would read the letter to let the audience know he couldn't make it because he's knee deep in the search for the Fountain of Youth or a treasure at the bottom of the sea or uncovering ancient Egyptian artifacts in the pyramids. It was a great concept, and we were excited to launch this idea the following year.

Through this entire process, I was continually keeping in contact with David Price, a great friend from Portland who calls to simply cheer me up. Knowing I was in pain, he recommended Dr. Smeltzer, a Theophostic counselor in Dallas, Texas. David always has a long list of people I should be meeting with or topics I should be thinking about, but I was interested in this counselor because of this term: Theophostics. *Theophostics* means to combine psychological processes with spirituality instead of choosing one versus the another. It seemed like an honest way to address actual problems, so I ended up buying a ticket to go down to Dallas, Texas for a full week before Christmas, 2012.

When I arrived, I stayed with Creighton, one of my all-time best friends I attended high school with. We immediately connected when he moved from Texas to Nebraska during our eighth-grade year. I remember how his Texas accent wooed the ladies, while I cursed my stars for the loss of the British accent I grew up with. Creighton introduced me to his kids, took me for a meal of solid Texas barbecue, went to a Dallas Cowboys football game with me and, knowing the guy who worked at a radio station, "won" us reclining leather seats near the court for a Mavericks game. It was quite the warm welcome to Texas.

When Monday came, I went to Dr. Smeltzer's office at his home in the suburbs. We had four-hour sessions for five days in a row. After each session I would leave and read through the material he had given me for that night. I truly appreciated his process as he dug down deep to deal with issues in me. Each day we got deeper and deeper into my issues that usually ended up circling back toward my relationship with Amy.

On the last day, Dr. Smeltzer asked if he could speak into my life with the Lord's leading. After counseling me for a full week, he wanted to pass along what the Lord had given him to say to me. I gladly agreed to this. For each patient, Dr. Smeltzer's message is shared using a clock, a structure used to deliver the twelve points he covers. And each hour of the clock has a different theme. For my buddy David Price, it was twelve cities around the world.

Dr. Smeltzer asked me to consider words of knowledge from my past, the present, as well as the future. I smiled as he put on his personally painted-over fake green Oakleys and leaned back in his chair. We sat in silence for several minutes before he began to talk. Finally, he spoke, telling me that God had given him landscape sceneries to serve as the backdrop for the twelve hours of my clock.

He began at 12:00, telling me about an image of a massive mining operation. There was a giant cliff, at the bottom of which there were excavators, dump trucks, and workers milling about. He told me he sensed the cliff was me, but my base was being mined out by these workers and this cliff was starting to crumble. Interesting. Back home I still stood tall in the public's eye just as this cliff was, but I never admitted my need for help. I imagine everyone around me thought I was taking this so well, both the cancer and the divorce, but internally, I was crumbling just as this giant cliff was about to do.

In the next scene, Dr. Smeltzer told me about a parade. And in one of the cars was Miss Texas, a five-foot eight-inch, beautiful blonde with blue eyes, who was waving to the crowd around her, seemingly the perfect picture of success and popularity. She was in a mint green jacket with a white blouse. He had absolutely no idea that his description perfectly described Amy, who'd been a top placer in the Miss Michigan competition. But inside of her, he could see the spirit of death and of rejection. He said that spirit was made up of complete evil and was attacking her. Now that, I connected with for Amy. I knew she was under attack from the enemy. This was starting to get interesting.

In the next scene, he told me about seeing a jungle scenario where animals were gathering. He saw an elephant and explained the meaning of how elephants never forget. This meant I had trouble forgetting my sins and was weighed down by the sin I felt from my past. That was totally true of me. I never actually let go of my past sins, despite having asked for forgiveness of them. Next, he told me he saw alligators. He said that represented a spirit that undermines masculinity and confidence. Well, that was obvious. My entire relationship with Amy's church was an attack on my masculinity as they tried to beat me over the head regarding my supposed issues with women in power.

Then he told me about seeing a praying mantis, which was symbolic of the spirit. What he didn't know is that the only thing on this planet my mother is deathly afraid of is a praying mantis. He talked about how this spirit was of fear and its capacity to affect me. That perfectly described my mother. I know, after spending hours and hours in hospitals, my mother carries a deep spirit of worry. As much as she loves me, she was always fearful of what the doctors said and always leaning toward worst-case scenarios in order to, I imagine, protect herself. Her opinion has great effect on me, and I knew this praying mantis was a sign for her and our future together.

The next scene was me sitting at the bottom of the ocean with unknown creatures swimming about me. This was hard for me to connect with in my own reality. But maybe it was evidence of me drowning at rock bottom? I was determined I would keep my eyes open; maybe something coming along in the future could be represented by this.

Next, he told me of a giant green field filled with beautiful purple and yellow flowers, looking as though it were a painting by a master painter. But in this incredible pasture were tiny wooden sticks coming out of the ground. Each of the numerous sticks had a tiny sign attached to the top of it. And every single one of them said, "N/A" or "Not Available." He knew these sticks were things that hadn't happened yet, but they were good things. He thought this was fascinating. It seemed that God had given him this vision, but had chosen to keep the details for Himself.

And finally, he told me the image he was receiving for the last hour was the simple image of a hand holding a smoking semi-automatic pistol. That was it. The room got quiet, and we both wondered what this meant. I asked if he had any more information. Was is symbolic? Was it literal? Am I going to die because of a someone else's handgun? Suicide? No answers.

He went on to describe my heart as a beautiful opera house. All of the rows and boxes were filled, and on the stage angels were singing the Hallelujah chorus. Then he noticed the building's ceiling was starting to crack, looking as though it was about to start crumbling, similar to the rock cliff. Ugh, that was me to a tee. I was holding onto myself and my reality for as long as I could before everything started crumbling down around me. I felt as though my heart was starting to fail.

Then he began telling me about walking through my soul and entering my spiritual heart. It was all very lovely imagery. Again, he made mention of an elderly woman, the exact same size and hair color of my grandmother who had just recently passed away. He told me she was praying fervently for me. And strangely enough, in that moment I could feel her presence all around me.

Overall, it seemed the majority of what he had to say came from Southern scenery. He had no idea my entire family was from the South, but he even suggested several scenarios with plantation farms filled with beautiful scenery and flowering trees. He mentioned horse racing several times. He talked about a generation full of dashed dreams, which I know related to my granddaddy from Tennessee. My granddaddy had created a new and innovative type of screw, but a business partner ended up stealing the plans and selling them for millions of dollars, while my mother's family suffered through overwhelming poverty in the tobacco fields of the South. I still have those same original screws in my writing desk to remind me of my past.

He told me that 2013 would be a year full of freedom and the day December 7th carried a very special meaning for me. It was all so fascinating, and I wish I could have brought a voice recorder so I could listen to it all again. But honestly, was I only listening to the words he was saying because they were kind? Sure, they seemed to be accurate, and I appreciated the fact he didn't paint me as a horrible person. But still, I winced at the idea that I paid money to be counseled and ended up listening to more prophecies. Was I just moving from one circus to another? But this, as well as every other prophetic word spoken, would be tested by time. I only hoped he was better at it than the crazy church Amy was still attending.

I remember the most interesting thing he had to say was about getting to the root of the difficulties between Amy and I. He told me I seemed to be missing the capacity to create "permanent bonds" in my life. I sighed when he said those words, immediately knowing he was spot on. My father and I also experienced this trouble as he raised me. The natural father-son bond was completely broken early on, which set the stage for all my relationships for the rest of my life. My relationship with him taught me to never trust an adult with specific, sensitive information, because later it would be turned and used against me in emotional manipulation. I felt the only adult figure I could trust was my mother.

I believe this was relevant to the issues that Amy and I were experiencing as well. Dr. Smeltzer asked if I had ever formed a permanent bond with her. I thought I had. But her recent behavior suggested that maybe I hadn't. Amy kept saying I was holding things back from her, but I knew I wasn't, or thought I knew. Was I fooling myself? My conversations with Dr. Smeltzer posed questions I simply didn't know the answers to.

I'll never forget one of the writings he sent me home with. Entitled "On Being Ordinary," this article was written to call out those who believed they were more than they actually are. And my word, this writing hit home. I knew this was me. I felt, in fact, that it was pointed at my entire generation. We were so focused on being "the best we could be" that we had lost sight of the long-term goals for our actual happiness. Dr. Smeltzer was asking me to be ordinary by forgetting my generation's grandiose search for worldwide popularity and perfection, so I could finally find peace. I was dumbfounded at both its simplicity and its profound impact on me.

Deep down, it resonated with me that what I honestly needed in my life was to "be ordinary." I grew up thinking, even being told by my parents, that I was unique and would win at everything I put my efforts toward. I realize now, looking back, that I was obsessed with being special; I was indeed convinced I could and should win. But I hated this idea that maybe, just maybe, I wasn't truly "set apart."

Before my meeting with Dr. Smeltzer, I read a well-researched article by McCann Worldgroup, "The Truth About Youth," which compiled more than 7,000 interviews with people from multiple countries declaring that Millennials were obsessed with three things:

> 1. Authenticity: the need to see things as they truly are.
>
> 2. Community: the need for connections and relationships.
>
> 3. Justice: the need for social or personal justice, to do what's right, to become an activist.

I saw how each of these three things had been so deeply ingrained in me and my friends, by the way we had been raised. I saw how, even from an early age, I became a great adapter, always searching for different areas where I could show off my authenticity and create better communications. I grew up being told I should take part in the movement for social justice. It was reinforced in me over and over that I could become a better person by giving to those in need.

But above all else, my personal desire was for true authenticity. I grew up with that idea in the forefront of my mind. This is why it was so special for me to finally share the story of my struggle with cancer with those I had been speaking to. As I traveled, I developed habits to show my authentic self, while discovering new and clever ways to protect who I actually was. I became ridiculously good at this. People would pat me on the back, saying how open and authentic I was, and such a great communicator. But all the while, honestly, I was only planning a new career of speaking about my cancer.

This concept of being ordinary brought back painful memories of my teen years.

When I was growing up, my family would ask me to hang out with them or stay home for a night, and I would semi-agree. I wanted to keep all of my options open just in case something better came up. I was a social climber, barely dedicated to anyone around me but fooling everyone by telling and showing them I was. I was good at tricking people. Maybe I should have pursued that acting career after all.

My sister, Angie, went so far as to label this lifelong behavior of mine as Wenzel-ing: "The act of holding onto all plans for as long as possible before finding the best plan to pursue." Maybe my habit of Wenzel-ing is why my family is constantly looking sidelong at me because I'm typically responding to a tweet, updating my Facebook status, or posting another Instagram photo.

Have I ever actually had an honest, truthful relationship? Or was I simply looking for my next relational high? Of course, I hated the idea that this concept could potentially exist inside of me. I despised it, but was this the truth? Was I, a Millennial, so dedicated to sharing my authentic story, communicating via social media, and giving to those in need, doing it all solely for my own benefit? Am I a real person or the culmination of everything I've seen that works, wrapped up into a blonde-haired, blue-eyed American boy?

Dr. Smeltzer told me I have an honest heart, but I seriously doubted it, because I could no longer feel it beating inside of me. I barely knew if my heart actually existed. His idea was to fix this type of mindset. He wanted me to focus "on being ordinary" and to fight against my concept of always being in first place, being the best of the best. I was to quit "Wenzel-ing" and following the self-prescribed rules for success I had set up for myself. But with these changes, I had absolutely no idea what my life could potentially look like. What if I allowed myself to become ordinary?

"I'm not being disobedient, I'm just following my dreams!" I overheard my little niece Lily say this six years ago, and it continues to haunt me. I had created so many dreams for myself, so many idealistic images I had to measure up to in order to give my life true meaning. I had been told my entire life that I am special and have a unique gift to offer the world. But what if the Millennial Generation, all eighty million— the largest generation of all time—had a similar carrot of heightened, idealistic expectation dangled in front of us and failed, just like I did? And worst of all, what if the pursuit of our entire generation to "follow our dreams" is actually the main source of our disobedience?

I love Peter Pan. Or at least I did, until I discovered why. I had recently come across an article discussing Peter Pan Syndrome. Peter Pan Syndrome isn't an actual diagnosis, but a pop-psychology concept of an adult (usually male) who is socially immature. The main issue with Peter is that he never had to grow up. Peter Pan represents *puer aeternus*, which is Latin for "eternal boy." He was never responsible for anything. He was the first to the party and the last to leave. He flew through life via fairy dust on his good looks and got whatever he wanted every single time. Other sources describe the syndrome further as, "coveting independence and freedom, chafing at boundaries and limits, and tending to find any restriction intolerable." I fear that I, as well as many in the Millennial Generation, have essentially become the Peter Pan Generation.

Humbelina Robles Ortega, a professor in the Department of Personality, Evaluation, and Psychological Treatment at the University of Granada, warns the overprotection of parents can lead children to develop this syndrome, given that "it usually affects dependent people who have been overprotected by their families and haven't developed the necessary skills to confront life. The 'Peter Pans' of present society see the adult world as very problematic and glorify adolescence, which is why they want to stay in that state of privilege."

Ann Yeoman, writer of *Now or Neverland: Peter Pan and the Myth of Eternal Youth*, ends her book with the idea that the internet has become our Neverland, providing us with our pixie dust, letting us fly away from reality, deeper and deeper into our own digital fantasies.

Peter refused to grow up and to meet the challenges of his life face on, waiting instead for his ship to come in and solve all his problems. Becoming Peter Pan was focused on feeding the fantasy that sometime in the future, the real thing, the most popular thing, the most profitable thing, would show up and save him. It becomes obvious that the one true fear for anyone suffering from Peter Pan Syndrome is to be eternally bound to anything or anyone of lesser value. Essentially, they become prone to "Wenzel-ing."

Humbelina Robles Ortega goes on to declare these people are scared of loneliness, which is why they attempt to continually surround themselves with people who can meet their needs: "They become anxious when they are evaluated by their work colleagues or their superiors, given they are completely intolerant toward any criticism. Sometimes they can have serious adaptation problems at work or in personal relationships." It's frightening to see that word "loneliness," considering it was the McCann Worldwide Advertising Agency who reported the Millennial Generation—the Peter Pan Generation—as "the largest generation to suffer from loneliness."

For Peter, the adventures always continue, but in reality, as we grow, we have to find a job, make car payments, pay our rent, buy food, and finish our taxes. In considering the idea that I was suffering from Peter Pan Syndrome, I was scared shitless. Becoming a responsible adult, capable of having adult conversations (as opposed to leading a crew of Lost Boys similar to me) was a frightening idea. Peter never had to grow up, but I did.

"Responsibility" is a horrific word to me. I worry that in my efforts to run from my early childhood memories regarding specific people in my life, I learned to pursue fun and excitement exclusively. I was afraid that Dr. Smeltzer was right and maybe I was a Lost Boy. And if I was truly incapable of making permanent bonds, I was essentially signing up to fly behind Peter Pan as he led us to the second star on the right and straight on till morning in order to reach my never-never land.

The acceptance of this massive negative concept overtook me. The trip to Texas was good overall, but it had introduced me to this issue I feared to face. But instead of trying to work through it by writing, or continuing counseling, I simply threw in the towel. In the weeks that followed, I quit caring about being authentic. I no longer cared about communicating. I stopped giving money to kids who needed chairs or kids dying from basic human needs like clean water. I had become so inwardly focused I barely noticed anything around me anymore. I gave up.

Maybe it was the finalization of the divorce, or maybe it was a summer of traveling where I was responsible for next to nothing. But when I got home to Grand Rapids, I had a horrible sense of unease about my future. So, to soothe that pain, I went to a car dealer, sprinkling my fairy dust all the way, and purchased my perfectly designed dream car: a smoke gray BMW 325xi. As a Lost Boy, I preferred not to "commute," but to dance and sing along with the words of J.M. Barrie's Peter Pan: "I don't ever want to be a man. I always want to be a little boy and to have fun."

SEVENTEEN
BEACHES SANS WATER

AFTER THE NEW YEAR, the words of Dr. Smeltzer were still ringing in my ears. When considering our time together, I felt both validated and undermined. He validated my conclusion that my relationship with Degeneration Church had been completely wrong and it was good to get out of there; validated the fact that although Amy had turned toward a new direction of her life, that didn't mean I had to follow her; and validated that I was still me, a whole person, and a valuable person to myself, my family, and to my God. Actually, saying and agreeing with those statements meant so much to me because it felt as if in the past year God had completely turned on me. But I was still undermined by the fact that I seemed to have a problem forming "permanent bonds" with others and that, quite possibly, I may have turned into Peter Pan.

I was now back in Grand Rapids, living with Heather and Michael. They were such dears to me. They let me move a bed into their spare room and gave me half of their other room to use as my office. I'm not sure what would have happened to me if Heather and Michael weren't a part of my life. It was so comforting to have them by my side as I entered hospitals and exited marriages. Deep down, I felt that sibling closeness to Heather, whether or not I said it to her. So, when I came back from Texas, it became my intention to develop a "permanent bond" with her.

I set up my office in their spare bedroom. I wanted this move to serve as my official restarting moment. Coming out of a year of divorce, I badly wanted to start over. And when I finalized the placement of my desk next to the window where I would accomplish my work, where I would write my letters, where I would pay my bills, I knew I had a chance to start over.

First off, I started regularly attending church with Heather and Michael. They had been going to The Vineyard church. Entering a church after a year like mine was one thing, but upon arrival, being freely offered grace and hope was nearly too much for me. I remember my first time there. I cried. I couldn't stop. And in the weeks that followed, during the worship music, during the sermons, during the offering, I just continued weeping. It had been so long since I tangibly felt God's love around me. And this church provided it. No more fake religion, just real, honest spirituality; pastors and people finally admitting their faults, their failures. Finally, no more perfect people.

I started off the year attempting to focus on my clients and began by working on a personality test for Erik Wahl, one of my favorite clients. I love to come up with new projects for my clients. I created a project called "The Artwork Revolution." I felt good because I was finally creating again. I was developing something that had never been developed. And the creation of something new is extremely exciting to me. Erik loved it, but we both knew it would be expensive. My payments were quick and steep.

But after agreeing with Amy to pay off my half of our credit card debt, she sent me an email asking me to pay $12,500 in thirty days. I remember looking at this bill and knowing, with every ounce of me, there was absolutely no way I could have ever paid this bill unless I was working on Erik's project. This single moment was even more evidence that God was somehow guiding and protecting me through this horrible process. He provided me with this absurd amount of money when I had absolutely none. Most likely to Amy's surprise, I paid her bill on time. But, my goodness, it hurt to write that check.

It could have been the pain of losing everything that was haunting me, but nevertheless my tumor continued to flaunt its power over me. On multiple occasions, I remember typing as my next partial seizure came on. When this happened, I realized I couldn't recognize the letters on my keyboard anymore. My brain knew I needed to type the letter "R," but while looking at the keyboard I couldn't tell which letter was which. So, I closed my eyes and thought hard about what the letter "R" looks like and started at the top-left side of my keyboard. 1?

Nope. 2? Nope. 3? Nope. I would strain myself, focusing on each of the keys until I found the letter "R." But before I could make it to the second or third letter the familiarity of the keyboard came back to me. I had no idea why I wouldn't just stop, close my eyes and recover. Maybe I felt like making that decision to rest meant the tumor had won that round, but I refused to let this bastard brain tumor win anything.

Back at The Sparrows, Lori was moving forward with the Creative Youth Center. We would propose our Captain H. Tanny's idea to our nonprofit backers and ask for their help to fund this new concept. We planned a fundraising event that Lori asked me to host. I loved it. Again, I was focusing on a project that meant something to me and used my skills as a communicator. I put together my speech and delivered it, using my presentation to describe how our nonprofit would be different from others in town. I explained how everyone in that room had parents who loved them and provided for them, so it was our duty to stand up for kids who never had that privilege. I pushed all the right buttons and pulled all the right strings. I had people coming up to me afterwards telling me they were in tears. It was a great event, and the nonprofit was moving forward with such enthusiasm that it felt great to be helping and creating again.

My conversations with Lori became frequent as we were driving around town. They moved from being business focused to discussing relational issues. I asked about her divorce from her husband, and Lori told me the truth. She told me about how their marriage broke down, about how the divorce process went, and what it was like afterwards. I remember once, as we pulled up in front of the CYC, she explained to me that the first person I dated after a divorce is always a bust. She predicted I would be so broken, so beat up, that my next relationship would definitely fail, and she told me I should be fully prepared for that. She went on to tell me about her first relationship post-marriage, how bad she felt moving on, and how that feeling made her next relationship a complete failure.

Somehow, I knew that would be the case with me. But through these ongoing conversations, I noticed that Lori had a crush on me. Not because I noticed how she was gently rubbing her neck while talking to me or tilting her head while smiling, but because she flat out told me. She told me that over the past six years, every time I walked into her coffee shop, her schoolgirl crush on me would grow. She relayed how nervous I made her each time I ordered. I felt bad. I hadn't even known her name until a few months ago! But Lori kept pressing. She was convinced of her feelings for me and didn't back down. I reminded her that she'd said the first relationship never worked out. She laughed and didn't know how to respond. She was interested, but I knew I couldn't pursue her. She was quickly becoming a great friend, not a girlfriend. I was having conversations with her that I wish I could have been having with my guy friends, but I didn't know any guys who had been through a divorce. She was my only source of wisdom.

In the meantime, my friend Jay and I had been dreaming of a trip where I would visit him in the United Arab Emirates. Jay worked with Leo A. Daly, a massive architecture firm in Omaha that was considering opening another office in the Middle East, so Jay and his family moved to Saudi Arabia for two years to do some initial business development. Jay created a plan to invite Brent and his girlfriend and me to visit. It started out as one of those plans you make at a bar late at night, but for some reason this trip was actually happening.

I bought a plane ticket for April 7th, 2012, to leave Detroit for Amsterdam, where I'd switch planes to Dubai. On the flight to Amsterdam, I knew the food would never match my diet. Everyone knows about plane food, but everyone also knows that we all succumb to it. And sure enough, at that moment of decision, when the beautiful, blonde stewardess with the incredible Dutch accent asked me if I wanted dinner, I said yes. It was pasta. I ate it.

Soon I realized my stomach had erupted into a riot. I couldn't even remember the last time I'd eaten pasta. I was sitting in the window seat next to two doctors who were discussing a case. I considered telling them that I needed help but was too embarrassed to bring it up. I looked around, seeing if anyone else felt sick. Nope. My pain and agony were growing. I couldn't believe this was happening. Typically, I never get sick when eating something abnormal. But I started getting warm, started feeling the tingling down the right side of my body. I asked the two doctors if I could scoot past them. I didn't want to have a seizure next to them, despite the fact they were the best possible seat partners for that scenario. I stumbled forward into the bathroom and locked the door behind me. I sat down on the closed toilet, put my head between my knees, as the heat in my body grew. The noise of the jet engines started spinning around in my head and I passed out.

I suppose if you were to have a seizure anywhere, the bathroom on an airplane would be a pretty great place. It's not big enough to actually fall to the floor, considering you're jammed in there. I honestly don't know if I had a seizure or not. I had no idea how long I was passed out. But eventually I woke up, having no clue where I was. It took me a few moments to realize I was in the bathroom of an airplane soaring at 35,000 feet above the Atlantic Ocean. But I felt slightly better. I exited the bathroom concerned everyone would be looking at me for being in there over an hour, but you can't see those glances when you refuse to look anyone in the eye. I stood for as long as I could next to the bathroom, probably several hours, just in case it happened again. I couldn't imagine squeezing my body back into my window seat. My stomach was still in intense pain, and my headache was worsening.

When we arrived in Amsterdam, I had a seven-hour layover. I was still in incredible pain and desperately needed to use the bathroom. I went to the airport hotel in the terminal and booked a room for my seven-hour layover. I went into the room and fell onto the bed to sleep for an hour and a half. When I woke, I stumbled to the bathroom and emptied my guts into the toilet. Then I pulled myself together and returned to the bed for another hour and a half, then went back to the toilet to vacate my body again. Back and forth. Back and forth. Those seven hours in Amsterdam were the most miserable I have ever experienced. My body was either in deep sleep or in deep evacuation, but when I left that room before my flight, I felt like an entirely new man.

The time I spent in Dubai and Abu Dhabi was incredible. We toured mosques, went to the top of Burj Khalifa (the tallest building in the world), ate incredible food (and poured through twenty bottles of wine in a week), and went on a dune buggy trip where we ended up lost in the Arabian desert. In our attempt to find our way home, listening to Guns N' Roses on full blast, we blew a tire only to discover our driver had failed to bring a spare. Who forgets to bring a spare when you are entering the desert? We had to call for help on a GPS phone, which led to more antics and another blown tire before we made it back. But being with my lifelong friends, it didn't matter whether I was lost or sick. It was just so good to be by their sides.

On my flight home, I determined to use my layover to visit the city of Amsterdam. It was about six in the morning when I wandered through the streets that still smelled like booze and bad decisions. But as I walked across the canals, I felt alive again. I went to a coffee shop, sat down, and wrote about everything that happened on my trip to Dubai. And when I returned to my new home at my sister's, I felt full of life and love.

Later that spring, I got an ecstatic phone call from Lori. The Kellogg Center had granted the CYC $250,000 in funding over the next three years. They were planning to throw a party, and she insisted I come as well. I joined them for a few drinks at the Meanwhile, before we switched locations to Kale's Corner, a bar on the Westside where karaoke is a staple. Never one to turn down a karaoke party, I joined. And the drinks just kept on coming.

Lori was a horrible karaoke singer, but she never turned down a chance to sing. I loved that. Amy was an incredible singer, but due to events earlier in her life with previous boyfriends, she never sang. She even sang for her Miss Michigan competition, which landed her in the top five, but that was before I knew her. I had never even actually heard her sing in church or along with the radio. But Lori sang "Fergalicious" like she wrote it. That's the type of girl I wanted in my life: a confident one, capable of not caring what her voice sounded like but excited to be in a bar with her dear friends as we all sang our hearts out.

I had a list of karaoke go-tos on my phone. I know that when I get a few drinks in me, I can never remember the best songs. First, I sang my go-to by The Darkness, "I Believe in a Thing Called Love," before I moved onto my dark horse, "Laid" by James. The songs went around the room again one more time before it got back to me. Lori told me she wanted to sing with me, so I checked my phone and saw the perfect song: "Don't You Want Me" by The Human League. I asked Lori if she knew it. She looked at me if I were crazy. Of course she did. This girl knows her 80s hits.

We went up there and belted it out. In tune, out of tune, it didn't even matter anymore. We stuck around, laughing and drinking, and I couldn't help but notice how much Lori seemed to love her life. She was running a successful coffee shop, starting a nonprofit organization for at-risk children, drinking in a bar with her dear friends and her brother, while crushing on me the entire time.

When the night was over, everyone was getting ready to head home. Lori's apartment was about three blocks from the karaoke bar, but like a gentleman, I offered her a ride home. We laughed all the way to the car, repeating songs, and recalling memories of this incredible night of celebration. As we pulled up to the front door of her condo, she reached behind me and began stroking my neck, "Keep driving." I went into silent mental shock. I knew exactly where this was headed.

"Where?" I asked.

"I don't care. Just keep driving," she answered.

No other spots were open and this night was remarkably warm, so we headed toward the beach. On the way there, my mind was in high speed. I needed to protect my heart, but there was something so fun about throwing all caution to the wind and letting the night fly away to wherever it wanted to go.

On the way, I started to spill more and more of my story. Of how things had fallen apart with Amy, of how hurt I was, of how painfully things had ended. Then, I most likely lied when I started sharing my hopes for my unknown future. I had absolutely no idea what they were. And mid-story we were interrupted by an 80s song on the radio, so we reverted to our karaoke section of the night. Forty-five minutes later we pulled up to an empty, pitch black beach. Sitting in the car, I told her about my first visit to the lake in college. Three of my friends and I drove up to Lake Michigan in October. And I remember demanding my first swim in this massive lake would be completely stark naked. I was slightly concerned this trip might follow suit (or no suit).

We got out and moved down to the beach. Without consent she cuddled close to me, and without consent I put my arm around her as she told me about her family, her six brothers, and how they felt both close and distant from each other. She explained why she ended up in Michigan and how The Sparrows was started with her ex-husband. She explained that when they divorced, he told her he would shut down the store, so she offered to take full ownership and run it. But when she did, she discovered he never actually paid any of the annual taxes. So, she spent the next several years paying down the store's $60,000 worth of tax debt. We talked more about the CYC and her hopes for her future there. But the conversation turned personal when she told me about her desire to have children with her ex-husband and the doctors told her it would never happen. The discussions became even more intense as she steered it closer toward her strong feelings for me. I felt horrible. I liked her, but wasn't sure this was the right time or if she was the right person. I hadn't kissed another girl since my marriage, and I was so nervous. Was I even a good kisser? I had absolutely no idea. But maybe this was a good thing. Secretly, I hoped Lori was drunk enough that she wouldn't remember all this awkwardness tomorrow.

In that tense moment, we heard a loud noise behind us and I jumped up to check it out. It was coming from the road. I had parked illegally and was concerned it could be a tow-truck in the middle of the night. We couldn't see the road because of the sand berms, so I used this as an opportunity to get out of this situation. I grabbed Lori and we started running toward the road. This was my chance to end this night before anything serious was started.

I got to the road to see there was nothing there. Lori asked me to go back down to the beach again. But I was eyeing my car. *This is it. You know exactly what will happen if you go back down to that beach.*

And it was then, maybe from the drinks or maybe from my overwhelming sadness, I turned around and followed her back down to the beach.

As we were walking she saw a beach chair and told me to sit in it. I did. Then she sat on my lap, looked me in the eyes, and held my face in her hands. I knew, one way or another, this moment would eventually happen. But I felt the deep pain of kissing another girl. Like it was an official death for Amy and me. Despite how Amy had treated me, despite the pain of the divorce, despite the situation with our personal items, I still felt bad kissing Lori. But nevertheless, we proceeded.

I felt new lips and new hips. New motions never felt before. New patterns of kissing I'd forgotten about. She put her hands on my back where Amy never did. She was focused on that lip, the opposite of Amy's preference. Her face felt different. Her runner's legs squeezed me. Her hands felt rough as they swept across my face. I realized she had spent years using and abusing her hands in the coffee shop, which were so different from Amy's delicate Photoshop hands. That first kiss was a conviction, a confession, and an offering of forgiveness all at once. We made out for a bit before we returned to the car and drove back home.

In bed that night, I didn't know what to think. It was Lori who told me that the first relationship after a divorce was always a letdown. Seems she was moving quickly, if she actually believed that.

All through this, I was so appreciative of Heather and Michael allowing me to stay at their house. Even though I wasn't telling them everything that happened with Lori, having the opportunity to spend time with my family each night was a comfort. One evening, I was in kitchen when I heard the doorbell ring. I went to get it and it was our dear friends, Seth and Sally. We started chatting, as I assumed they were there to meet Heather and Michael for dinner. I offered Seth a beer and then the doorbell rang again. It was Micah. That's strange. I offered him a beer as well, but then the doorbell rang again. It was Chuck and Holly. Wait a second. Something is going on here.

Eventually, the house was filled with my closest friends, and I was in complete shock as to what was going on. In the middle of my conversations I tried to calculate my half-birthday. Nope. Was it a National Cancer Day? National Divorce day? Nope. I was standing in the kitchen, laughing at how odd this was, when Heather piped up with a message from the group of twenty or so people. She told me that she, as well as the rest of the room, were all proud of me, that I had handled the divorce well, even to the point of giving up everything I owned to create peace with Amy.

She told me she had gathered up all of my friends and asked for donations to purchase me my own white Herman Miller Eames rocker, the piece of furniture I hated parting with the most when I took everything back to Amy's house. She pulled it from around the corner, and I was in complete shock. I couldn't believe what Heather and Michael had just done. I sat down in the middle of the kitchen in my new white rocker just beaming with pleasure. I'm sure I ended up giving some type of off-the-cuff speech, but in the back of my mind I vividly remembered my previous year, while living in my temporary apartment. It appeared Heather had essentially read my mind as I was dreaming of "that" chair, the one that could be purchased for a refugee, for a victim, for a retiree, that would show them that somebody cared, that someone had prepared a place for them to sit down and experience love and peace. Heather and Michael, as well as the rest of my family and friends, had all welcomed me and given me my own chair to rest and recover in.

That chair, to this day, is the best gift I have ever received.

EIGHTEEN
A GLASS OF BOURBON, A FORWARD WOMAN

BECOMING A REGULAR at the weekly dance parties at Rocky's isn't necessarily something you would want to write home about. I always knew I could never dance, but whiskey had its own thoughts on that matter. The majority of weekend nights, my friends and I would pack into the top floor at Rocky's, and I'd drink enough to forget. At the end of these nights, we would all end up climbing on top of the bar, our filthy, hooch-covered fingers digging into the dirty and crumbling ceiling. Miraculously, the bar held our combined weight as we leaned out over the bouncing crowd, belting out the last song of the night at the top of our lungs, "All My Friends" by LCD Soundsystem:

You spent the first five years trying to get with the plan

And the next five years trying to be with your friends again

You're talking 45 turns just as fast as you can

Yeah, I know it gets tired, but it's better when we pretend

It comes apart, the way it does in bad films

Except in parts, when the moral kicks in.

I wouldn't trade one stupid decision

For another five years of life

If I could see all my friends tonight.

If I could see all my friends tonight.

If I could see all my friends tonight.

Speaking of "friends," one night I saw Lori across the dance floor, but this time she looked so much different. She looked beautiful in this light. And by light, I mean bass-driven flashes of color and visible sound shaking the room. It was good to see another person who had gone through all the same shit I had. We probably should have shut down that party and told the young kids to go home and prepare for their future which was about to destroy them. But instead, I turned around at the bar and, with my head in my hands, ordered another whiskey. There was no chance I would be able to drive myself home.

Lori waltzed over to me and slyly suggested I could stay at her place, the "Lion's Den," as I had come to call it. I knew it. I knew it right there on that dance floor that if I went with her I would have sex that night. Then a wispy, strange voice circled my ears and slowly entered my cancer-filled brain: *"David, what do you have? You have no furniture. You have no permanent place to live. You have no idea where your career is going. You're depressed. You have nothing, and cancer is going to kill you. Each day you wake up, deciding to throw caution to the wind, so why not now? Why can't you just enjoy this moment?"*

We stumbled the few blocks back to her condo. We stumbled into her room and we stumbled into sex. It was unpoetic, drunken, and blurry-eyed, but it was the first sex I'd had since my marriage. And from what I can piece together, it was quite mind-blowing. This act essentially freed me from Amy, but it also made me feel free from God. However, that type of freedom made me feel like I was all alone again.

Several days later, Lori and I met over a wonderful sushi lunch. I knew what this was about—a discussion about our night together. She asked how I felt, but I told her I couldn't feel anymore. I felt that I had left my body and was now watching it from afar. I started feeling so bad about what I had done with her that I began making even worse decisions.

That summer I succeeded in completely destroying my body. I had muscular pains from seizing and passing out in the bottom of the YMCA's shower, nearly unusable feet from the scratches and torn flesh from a tubing misadventure on the river, a black eye from drunkenly stumbling down a 10-foot rock cliff, sunburnt shoulders from Zac's bachelor party, massive bruises on the inside of my right leg from falling through a wooden dock, what felt like a broken rib from a firework-related incident when I got accidentally punched in the chest, a strained tendon in my foot after racing through the sky ramps downtown, and I seemed to have a broken butt bone from a slip in the driveway. But I knew how to clear all this pain up. More booze.

A few weeks later, Lori and I realized that our "event" had passed and we still wanted to be friends with each other. We went out to the beach in the hot Michigan weather to relax. But I found myself peeking as she removed her pants to reveal her toned runner's legs. I was hanging out with my dear friend who openly admits she wants me. And that was a pretty big thing for me at this point in my life. I loved to be wanted.

I had recently learned I have the personality type of being extremely social but never forward in relationships. I desire lust. Not to lust after, but to be lusted over. People with this type of personality never need to flirt with girls, because they put out the vibe that draws the interested girls toward them. Looking back, I can see why Lori was my best friend. She wanted me, and I loved that feeling of being wanted.

Lori and I continued going out to eat on the business credit card, talking about life, divorce, and the CYC. But I saw how an actual relationship with her would turn out. It looked like work, not romance. It looked like I would have to help her out at her coffee shop. It looked like I would serve as her number two at the CYC, driving around in her red Ford Fiesta. It looked like raising her dog and two cats who covered her messy condo in pet hair. That wasn't what I wanted. Lori was written into my life to serve as an amazing friend but never anything more.

One night, after dinner, Lori and I went for a drive. We ate dinner and ordered Maker's Mark whiskies while talking about work, which led to another bar where we ordered Maker's Mark whiskies to talk about life, which led to another bar where we ordered Maker's Mark whiskies to talk about divorce. Anchor Bar was the last place we visited and only a few blocks from her condo. We hung out there for a bit, putting on our own private karaoke show, before I drove her to her condo at Union Square on the Westside of town. We parked on the side of the road for me to drop her off. She, as always, asked me to come inside and I, as always, told her, "Nope, I'm sorry. Goodnight."

I was sitting in the driver's seat of my BMW when she started slowly taking off her pants. Dammit, she knew my weakness for her legs! Then she leaned across and started kissing my neck. I needed to just get out of there or I was going to make more bad decisions. I can't tell you how long we sat there, confessing, laughing, smiling. I felt bad sending her across the dark street to enter the overwhelming doors of her condo, which was inside an old high school building built in the early 1900s that looked like a castle. But I also thought it would get us out of the car and give us some space.

So, I asked her, if I walk her to the door, would she let me go? She agreed, so we got out of the car, looked both ways, and crossed the street to her condo. As I said goodnight, she leaned in and kissed me with serious intent. Then that similar co-pilot thought for the entire summer crossed my drunken mind: *"David, you have been screwed over. You were given cancer, your life is on the line, your wife rushed you through a shitty divorce, and now you are all alone. When you get back home, you will look back on this moment and curse yourself forever if you don't take action now."*

So, I did.

We rushed upstairs blasting through her front door, shirts flying, shoes being flipped off. It became a competition to see which hipster could get their skinny jeans off fast enough. Hands and arms were flailing, tearing off clothes as we fell down onto her bed. I told her I didn't have a condom and she looked at me strangely, reminding me it was impossible to get her pregnant. She quickly repeated the story, that after ten years of trying, it was impossible. I thought about that as I laid on my back looking up at her, with her hair cascading down all around my face. And somehow, in the back of my inebriated mind, that small specific voice that is so easily ignored told me it wouldn't be the same with us. Almost like a challenge set before me, I knew I had the power to get her pregnant, but I was too drunk to care.

I knew from previous conversations regarding her upbringing and former relationships that Lori had become an atheist. So, I asked her, in between kisses, that if I managed to get her pregnant would she believe in God again. She laughed and sarcastically replied with, "Sure." I looked at her with whatever conviction I had left in my drunken eyes, raising my voice and asking again, "Seriously! Will you?" She lowered her head, looked directly at me, and replied both whimsically and honestly, "Yes. Yes, I will."

NINETEEN
KINFOLK-ITIS

MY GET-OUT-OF-JAIL-FREE SPEECH TO LORI WAS PERFECT. Obviously, that night was a huge mistake and the relationship had to be stopped immediately. In fact, maybe it was time for me to leave my position at the CYC as well. She invited me to her friend's wedding in Montreal, but luckily, I had previous engagements. A wedding date seemed like an unspoken agreement that everything would be okay in the future, but I knew that it wouldn't. When she got back, I intended to sit her down for this speech I'd been planning. But one and a half weeks later, before I could get together the guts to set up this meeting, I got a text from Lori.

She wanted to grab dinner. But there was something mysterious about this text, almost as if the true meaning of it were displayed in hidden words beneath the actual images on my phone. I could tell *something* was up, so I asked her to call me immediately. My phone rang…

"David, today is a crazy day. It's my nephew Ryan's birthday, my dad just had a small stroke, and I'm having your baby."

Silence is a weak word to describe the emptiness, the blackness, the hollowness that followed that statement.

And then, the questions.

"Are you sure? Are you really, really sure? But what about the doctors who told you this wasn't even possible? You told me it was impossible for you to get pregnant!"

That was followed by a rather repetitive, curse-laden understanding of the news I'd received. Somewhere, I imagined, there was a drunken celebration party going on and my sperm were signing autographs. I agreed to meet for dinner, knowing it was my "parental duty" to take the next steps alongside her. We agreed to meet one hour later at Terra, a small restaurant in Eastown.

I don't know why, but as I drove to dinner I thought of Pastor Goldman. He was my childhood preacher at First Baptist Church in Papillion, Nebraska. And being a true Southern Baptist preacher, his voice sounded like a gravelly Harley Davidson motorcycle engine. And when he yelled, or—excuse me—when "the spirit moved in his soul," he simply revved up that engine. But now, his loud and pointed words were not focused on the sinners found on the streets, nor were they focused on the prisoners whose crimes had found them guilty. His voice was now focused on me. And I knew exactly how it would sound, "YOU ARE A DRUNKEN FORNICATOR!"

Lori and I sat across from each other in immeasurable silence. The pain and agony were equivalent to a break-up dinner. But this was the opposite. This was a together-forever dinner. This was a worlds-colliding dinner. This was the understanding-that-my-life-would-be-eternally-linked-to-her-life dinner. I had stumbled onto something bigger than cancer, something bigger than divorce. I was 50 percent responsible for a new human being that would show up sometime in (count it out on the fingers) May. After dinner, I knew I needed to escape. Again.

I had to keep talking, to explode with tears, frustration, and curse words. So, I called Micah and asked if I could come over. When I arrived, I realized my body felt actual physical damage, like an impact wound of some sort. This news had risen above emotional pain and become physical pain. When I arrived, Micah's warm hug reminded me he would never judge me for what I'd done. We went out into the back yard and he lit a fire. We sat around it as I explained my scenario, tears sliding down my face. I told him that I felt my life was over. But Micah, the trooper he is, listened, let me get it all out, and when my body was near passing out from exhaustion, simply told me that God still loved me, my family would still love me, my friends would still love me, and he still loved me.

Part of my frustration was that he was right. I would be forgiven, but only because

I *needed* forgiveness. I would be protected, but only because I *needed* protection. I would be surrounded by people, but only because I *needed* to be surrounded by people. And I'm not used to *needing* things. I'm not used to needing forgiveness, needing to be protected, needed to be surrounded by people. And then I thought of Amy. I had finally proven myself to be the lying, cheating, sleeping around type she always assumed me to be. I could no longer claim innocence to my friends and family.

That night, I lay in bed knowing that any public goodwill that had been built around me through this cancer and divorce would soon be forgotten. I would never be forgiven for knocking Lori up. I began building an argument with my would-be detractors: "Listen, this is my first and only one-night stand! This is not my typical behavior! This is not who I am! This is not what I do!" But apparently, it is who I am and it is what I do.

The next morning, I woke up feeling fantastic, remembering the misery of the dream I just had. But a split second after, I realized it was all backwards. It was my dream that told me this entire scenario was all a dream. It was my reality I had become so afraid and ashamed of.

Lori and I met nearly every single day from that point on. We would meet up to, if nothing else, sit across the table from each other. And eventually we had the idea, well, we can't hurt anything anymore. So, we started having sex again.

I get why sex addicts say having sex removes their pain for just a brief moment. It served as the best momentary relief from the pain each of us were going through. But I always ended back up in the same place of fear and disappointment in myself.

I was a mess at home. Part crying, part sniveling, seemingly lost as I ended up wandering between my home office five feet from my bedroom next door. I knew I had to tell Heather and Michael. So, one night, after dinner, we were sitting on the back porch. My stomach was doing intense somersaults as the truth bubbled up inside of me. Finally, with tears coming from my eyes, I told them that I had gotten Lori pregnant. Heather, like a good sister, gave me an embrace I knew only comes from sibling kindness.

Next, I had to tell my friends. At the end of September, we all went North on a wine trip. We moved from winery to winery before we ended up at the final location of the day, Brys Estates. We all had a bit too much to drink, and we found ourselves in our final tasting. With the weather starting to turn outside, we were all bundled up in our sweaters and knit hats, while conversations bounced back and forth and everyone was having the best time. In the middle of all this, I held up my glass for a toast. They looked at me strangely, then started yelling, "Toasts!" So, I breathed deep, and said, "A toast…to my new baby I'm having with Lori!" Jaws dropped and drinks were spilled as everyone circled and danced around me in a giant bear hug. Jill, Kate, and Caton, of course, started crying while Zac, Cameron, and Ben's mouths hung wide open as they started laughing. Carson looked quite dazed, but that was rather typical for him. It was so good to share this news with my friends, who I knew would love me through any mistake I made.

But as I returned home from that trip, to the silence of my borrowed bedroom, I realized I was sick. I was suffering from a case of Kinfolk-itis. Kinfolk is a Millennial magazine that has wrapped itself into the ethos of what it means to be young, crafty, beautiful, and to create everything at home using what you dug up from your garden in your country cottage. Kinfolk-itis was all about leaning forward into the best and most beautiful parts of life.

That's my disease: leaning. I leaned too far forward because I wanted *that* girl in *that* magazine. I wanted that dream of a girl, as opposed to an actual girl herself. I leaned forward in my desire as my body ached to walk into parties with a girl who knew how to act, who knew the popular things to say, who knew not to tell a compliment-payer she got half-off her outfit at Target. I realized I wanted my Tumblr girl: a simple image of something beautiful. But what did that say about me? Nothing good.

Lori made for a perfect best friend, the tomboy friend you'd have as a child, with whom you can talk about what you're afraid of, but seemed like she might be a horrible party-goer. Maybe that was the deep reason I couldn't accept her as that role of girlfriend in my life. At this point in my life, post-divorce, I didn't want a partner. I wanted the perfect date to the next perfect party, someone to keep my mind off my actual reality.

I fear my generation, the same generation that moved from drinking hose water to filtered water, has fallen prey to this new style of thinking; this horrible idea of marrying "Kinfolk girls." We grew up the prized children of financially strong Baby Boomers who watched over us, handling each of our needs with their deepest attention. They followed us to school, called the principal to suggest alternative ways to do things. They called our college professors to chew them out over our unjustly received grades. And we reacted to this freedom with absolutely no fear for our future. We wanted to help those around us. We wanted to be of service to others. We grew up focused on nonprofits. We wanted, more than anything, openness in our friendships, but realized we were still, like every other generation who came before us, scared. But then the internet opened up another line of communication, and we realized we could form our own online persona that had no connection to our offline personality.

I've concluded this deep inner feeling of needing to belong, yet fearing it at the same time, is the root of Kinfolk-itis. It perfectly captures those moments we all long for, we all strive for. I wanted my Lana Del Rey, my Carla Bruni, my Sienna Miller. *This* person was the one throwing her head back laughing as she passed another bottle of perfectly aged Napa Valley wine over the cups of homemade raspberry-mint tea, across the handmade wooden table in the candlelit backyard, underneath white lights hanging from flowering trees, next to the gardens filled with hearty vegetables like radishes and kale.

Brené Brown's research on social interaction has opened up this concept of true vulnerability. In a photo on Instagram or in a blog post, we "share," but we're not really sharing. Few are willing to truly share and risk their perfectly coiffed online image, and our sense of insecurity that has been slowly growing since the mid-90s. Over time, I fear Kinfolk-itis won't be too far from actual bipolar disorder. We develop our online personality in direct contrast to our offline personality. This generation, my generation, is all too prone to suffer from this new type of dual personality disorder. With all of our communication, openness, and "honest talk," we should be near the apex of generational maturity. So how on earth are we scientifically measured to be the loneliest generation on record?

But of course, due to our intense understanding of "others," we've become completely aware of this. We've realized how empty we feel, so now we must look at it and publicly name it, but that still has nothing to do with fixing it. We are all aware that the need to "be real" is increasing, but all that really does is pull the mask further over our heads. We claim we're being real, when all of us know we aren't. I succumb to this far too often. I write a post, I take a photo, and I share it. No harm there. But I, maybe like many of us, frequently come back to see the likes, read through the comments, subconsciously compare the likes to so-and-so's page, or maybe re-analyze my image for why the likes were so low.

We try so hard to be liked. We try so hard to type the right thing. We try so hard to show our "vulnerability" by displaying ourselves slightly bruised and battered, but never down and out. We slowly and perfectly dip our heads at life's struggles, then post a beautiful photo of a sunset or a city, or (my favorite) the shot out of an airplane window coupled with a quote of a Franciscan monk or an old foreign poet.

But what happens when you can't cover up your mistakes anymore? What actually happens when your world falls apart, and not in a Mumford & Sons way, but in an honest and true way, when you feel rock bottom has become your new bed partner? That's the question I had to ask, faced with the decision to tell Lori, this wonderful girl, that she simply didn't play into my perfect life. She had ruined the past years of carefully curating my public image, created through publicly and properly dealing with my cancer and my divorce, by taking what was given to me and forming it to my own advantage. But this pregnancy seemed nearly impossible to turn around for good. It was up to me to publicly eat crow, and no, that's not crow pâté nestled between leafy greens and roasted beets.

I called my sisters, admitting to them my horrendous error. Our "perfect family" had been damaged by my miserable action. Each of my two older sisters handled the news with such grace. They told me how much they loved me and this baby would be welcomed as a part of our family. I hate to say it, but I was floored by my family's response. More so, I was shocked at how everyone handled it with such an open heart of love toward me and Lori.

And now, the worst. I left Lori's apartment and walked through the rainy streets of Grand Rapids, crossing back and forth over the bridge stretching across the Grand River. I was soaked but didn't care. It was time to tell my parents that their baby boy had slept with some random girl and gotten her pregnant.

I told my parents that I had gotten Lori pregnant and winced as those words came out of my mouth. But again, my words were received with love and a firm commitment to love this baby as their own to the very end. Even through my misery, as I lay prostrate on the ground before them, my family told me to get back up and keep on walking.

Strangely enough, my mother somehow knew I had gotten a girl pregnant. She told me God had already began easing this idea into her head. She had met Lori earlier that summer on a trip to Grand Rapids. My mother, a lifelong librarian, sat down to talk to her about acquiring books for the Creative Youth Center. When Lori got up to refill our drinks, my mom turned and looked at me grinning, like we were in junior high, and asked if I was interested in her. No, I said. She wasn't my type. Nevertheless, my mother swears she could have stopped me before I dropped the bomb and predicted I had gotten Lori pregnant. I suppose that should stand as evidence of my mother trading in her motherly intuition for her motherly crystal ball.

In time, I knew people would recognize Lori's noticeably growing stomach and my noticeably stiffening jaw. Eventually, we'd have to share the news. So, on October 29th, I wrote a blog post titled, "So Then This Happened." It recalled my hesitations to share the news of who I had become. I shared in the first two paragraphs that I, a cancer ridden, recently divorced man, was about to become a father.

I was overwhelmed by excited people sharing their congratulations. Comment after comment was filled with joy and excitement for the two of us. I recall thinking to myself that, in the future, whenever anyone tells me they are surprised by a pregnancy, I should immediately respond with loud cheers of joy and big hugs. I knew this is what they would need, because it was exactly what I needed at this moment. So as a note to myself in the future, I promised to deliver that gift to them. I do remember a few painful comments of disapproval, one from a dear friend of mine. But Heather, my online protector, went after him and called him out to show grace in moments like these. I couldn't help but smile when I imagined my family circling their wagons around mine, with their shotguns locked and loaded for whoever came too close.

But no guns were drawn that day. I feel the admission of an unplanned pregnancy truly brought out the honest response Lori and I were desperately searching for. My friends and family knew this was never planned. They knew we were screwed. They knew we didn't have enough money to handle this. They knew us, and still, they loved us even more because (unwittingly) we had reminded them of what true authenticity and vulnerability looks like: to be ripped open in public shame with no excuses, with no clever poems or quotes to hide behind, to simply accept what happened as the truth, yet be asked to wake up again tomorrow and continually deal with the consequences of our actions.

I so badly wished I could have pushed pause and hesitated for eternity, but Lori's belly continued to grow like a strange countdown clock, ending previous stories and beginning new ones. I was being forced to take this unavoidable first step toward a future with a baby and a woman that came out of nowhere. Lori and I didn't know what to do next. This horrific news had become public and somehow, someway, we still felt loved.

Lori was smart enough to leave her condo she owned in order to make room for the baby. Her brother Todd, who I knew through the CYC, stepped in to make sure his younger sister had whatever she needed. He even fronted her a hefty amount of cash so as not to delay the move when she found a lovely house to rent in Eastown, as well as money to pay for the baby's birth. Lori moved into the house on Richard Terrace in December of 2013. I visited daily to help her set up her home, dealing with my ongoing tension as I realized this could potentially be my future home.

Lori was patient, yet eager to hear my prolonged response about what I was going to do next. Was I going to stick around and form a relationship with her? Or was I going to jet off to a faraway city and start my new Kinfolk life? And I determined that when we met at her new home, I would sit her down and have a conversation about our future.

On December 7th, I told her I wanted to be with her through and after this pregnancy. I wanted to be the father to our child and maybe, someday, some type of boyfriend or husband to her, while internally knowing I may have to do this with or without feelings for her. She deserved my presence, so maybe I could give it my best shot and be with her and our child for the rest of my short life. Whether this pregnancy was brought on by inebriation or not, my decision at that moment would serve as the final result of who I truly was. Knowing the intensity of this scenario, I dedicated myself to serve her and our new child. That, in the end, standing before God, this would be the biggest factor of how my life was spent on this earth.

At that time, I had forgotten it, but during my sessions with Dr. Smeltzer in Dallas, he had set aside a specific date that would be of great importance to me. I eagerly asked why, but he said he didn't know. That date was also lost within the "Not Available" signs in the image he had of that beautiful open field. Looking back at my journal, I realized that day was December 7th.

TWENTY
GOING HOME

I TRIED TO REMEMBER ALL OF THEM, but the lasting damage to the memory portion of my brain was so intense I couldn't remember their names, let alone place them on the correct individuals. That December I was to be introduced at the Slager household for a Christmas dinner, but more importantly, to Lori's six older brothers: John, Bill, Dean, Randy, Jeff, and Todd. They grew up in a construction family. The oldest, Jon, was seventeen years older and shared a birthday with Lori. Then the rest of them were spread out several years apart. These weren't just brothers. They were construction workers with scarred hands and hidden emotions, who made themselves known by the loudness of their voices. Lori wasn't entirely sure how they would handle me, the guy who knocked up their little sister.

Prior to showing up, I was given a preview of what to expect, as Lori explained her childhood, which included "Slager Fest." It was essentially what every parent is scared of when their kids entered high school. Slager Fest was a week-long beer-soaked party at their house while their parents were away on vacation for a month. When I think back on what it must have looked and sounded like, it seems more like an awesome college party movie. Kegs upon kegs were stacked up as the entire school gathered to partake in this debauchery. And little Lori, standing off to the side, was so proud of all of the friends her older brothers had.

But now, they were all married and had families full of the newest Slagers. There were sixteen grandkids whose names, accepting personal grace from myself, I didn't even try to remember. The oldest niece, Jen, was twenty-four, and the youngest, Luke, was three. They all lived within fifteen minutes of each other except her brother Todd, who also lived in Grand Rapids.

I met Lori's parents, John and Madeline. John was seventy-three and, from what I saw, had lived life down to the bone. He was nearly physically broken, having owned and managed the construction company that all of the brothers grew up working at. He was a large man who, despite having had several small strokes, was still drinking every day at a local bar. Lori had spent the last year explaining to me what it was like to grow up in this environment, watching as he came home and drunkenly dealt with his six unruly boys. After meeting John, I came to see him as his own massive planet, and the closest you could get to him was to satellite around him, never attempting to enter his atmosphere.

Lori's mother, Madeline, on the other hand, couldn't wait to meet me. She had known that Lori had a crush on me and, while this wasn't exactly the best scenario, we were in this together and that made her happy. In the past few years, in order to deal with her husband, she had become deeply entrenched in her faith as well. There were moments when she started asking me questions or making statements that sounded a little too much like Amy, but I knew she was harmless. She was a lovely woman who would do whatever she could to help us.

Later that evening, the entire family, nearly forty of them, were gathered in the house and everyone was looking at me out of the corner of their eyes. Me, this random guy who just knocked their sister up, their daughter, their aunt. Looking back, I really should have been much more scared, considering how little I knew of them. I only had a few details, the highlight being they were all Bears fans. And I knew enough about the Bears to hold a sturdy conversation. Lori laughed, saying that as soon as I shared a few details about the Bears' performance last Sunday, they all collectively shrugged and accepted me as part of the family.

We spent that night at the main Slager household that was filled with black-haired Chicagoans, with their strong accents and muffled curse words. Kids were running around attempting to interact with adults, or else sat in the corner messing with their phones. It was a beautiful circus. I had never had any honest interaction with my cousins. They were perfectly kind to me, but too old to play with. But here, there were sixteen kids all close in age and who looked so much alike it was difficult to place them with their actual parents. Lori and I had our photo taken, which today still stands on top of their fireplace. Lori, with a huge smile is pointing at her belly bump, while I'm standing behind her with a surprised look of "Oops, THAT happened!" I cringe each time I look at it, but I've come to learn that reality is often cringe worthy.

A few days after Christmas, we took a flight to Omaha where we would visit my parents. My three sisters had already met Lori at our ThanksChristmas celebration in November. For that trip, we traveled up to Mechanicsburg, Pennsylvania where my entire family had been very welcoming of her. I knew they would be, based on the previous conversations we had. But this trip to Omaha was more about her meeting my close friends. And of course, upon arrival into Omaha, my father drove us from the airport through downtown to show us the growing sculpture collection detailing the pioneers move to the West in their wagons, the geese, the ducks, and the buffaloes. I apologized to Lori, telling her he still takes me by these sculptures and explains them all every single time he picks me up at the airport.

That night, we went out to Jay's bar, where the drinks were free and the house music was loud. Later that night, we all ended back at Jay and Holly's house with Brent at our side. We gathered around his kitchen table as Jay took great pride in remembering our days of high school, sharing our memories, retelling stories from our time in the Middle East, while mind-blowing wine was passed around the table. I remember a moment in the midst of all of the noise and commotion, when Jay leaned in, looked at me, and said, "She's the one." I was shocked that Jay felt so certain about her. In celebration of my homecoming, we drank so much wine that night that Holly had to drive everyone home. But the whole way we refused to stop singing, yelling stories, and cackling. There is no better feeling than introducing a girl, a uniquely special girl, to your best friend and getting his stamp of approval.

When we arrived home that night, my parents had set up two separate bedrooms for Lori and me, but I was drunk as a sailor, so I smiled as I dragged her into my room to sleep in my bed. There is something strangely fulfilling, even at thirty-two, about giving the finger to your parents' plans and doing whatever the hell you want. The best part was the next morning when my dad stuck his head into my room to tell me something and saw a girl's head asleep next to mine. His eyes quickly averted mid-sentence as he popped back out. The fifteen-year-old hungover version of me grinned as I turned over and nuzzled up against Lori as I went back to sleep.

When we returned to Grand Rapids in January, I moved into the same house that Lori had begun renting the month before. Moving was a breeze. Everything was already boxed up, so it was moved directly to the attic. Of course, I had no furniture to offer her except for my new chair. But we were together and were able to sleep in the same bed. We were both so new to this situation that everything was filled with excitement. Is it a girl? A boy? She originally wanted to learn, but I refused to. I saw this surprise as our one true unknown gift. I told her she could learn, but then she'd have to spend the rest of the time hiding it from me because I didn't want to know. Knowing that was impossible, she agreed and we decided to learn the gender at birth.

We were learning all of this new baby talk together. One of the biggest development tools we learned was to play music for it. We would lay in bed for hours and cycle through songs including Beyoncé, Daft Punk, and Elvis. We determined that the baby loved the Honky-tonk beat considering it responded the most to Johnny Cash. My Tennessee ancestors would have been proud.

We were surrounded with love for our baby from our friends and our families. And that love wore off onto each other. I knew Lori had a crush on me, but that crush grew to honest love. And I, who months before had been so unsure, started to fall in love with her as well. Not only because she was carrying my unborn child, but because I finally saw how kind and giving she was to me. She was polite. She was a hard worker. She told me that she would take over all of the sleeping duties when the baby was born so I could get plenty of rest. I realized that Lori was a girl who would wake up early, work at her coffee shop, stay late at her nonprofit, and do it all while smiling as she served those around her. Lori has a heart full of love that she expresses both through her words, but also through her actions.

We were interested in having this baby at home as opposed to the hospital. While still getting checkups with a doctor (who happened to be a previous client of Amy's), we met with Yolanda from Birth Song. Her company was located in an office just around the corner from our home. She had home-delivered over 3,000 babies in the past thirty years and knew her stuff. It was interesting to see her interact with us. Maybe it was due to our scenario, but she seemed to focus exclusively on Lori and made only occasional references to me as she casually glanced my way. But I eventually weaseled my way into her heart. She was so kind, simply fantastic at her job, and Lori felt safe with her in this new experience. Yolanda explained the whole process as we listened to heartbeats, measured bellies, and learned what would happen the day the baby showed up.

Night after night we lay in bed next to each other coming up with names for both a girl and a boy. It was tough. We figured out a boy's name pretty quickly, but our girl name was giving us trouble. Then one-day Lori suggested a name and I was sold.

Everyone was convinced we were having a boy, and I considered that my fear, based on the uneasy relationship with my father, would be brought full circle by God. It was incredibly annoying when my father kept sending us emails about circumcision "due to our Jewish heritage." Madeline, Lori's mother agreed that Lori was carrying the baby the exact same way she carried her six boys. Even people walking past her in the grocery store or checking her belly out at the coffee shop would tell her, "You've having a boy." But Lori seemed to know something we didn't. Her maternal instincts kept telling her it was a girl.

Our musical tradition continued. Each night we would go through Lori's Spotify list, searching for a baby song that would fit the bill to play after our little one was born. We wanted something light, something catchy, something we wouldn't get sick of singing again and again. Then I remembered a song from Her, a futuristic movie directed by Spike Jonze, starring Joaquin Phoenix and Scarlett Johansson. The plot was focused on a computer program that formed human relationships and started to understand human behavior so well that it started to replace best friends and lovers. In the movie, "The Moon Song" serves as this special little song the main character and his digital lover share, singing it together late at night. We listened to it and immediately knew it was perfect. So, from that night on, we began and ended our musical explorations with that specific song and declared it would be our future bedtime song.

As the pregnancy progressed, Lori started telling me that the baby knew me. But I didn't understand what she was saying. She explained that when we were at a party or at Sparrows, whenever I came close, the baby could hear my voice and would start to roll around and kick. And when I left, it would stop. Lori explained to me that the baby knew my actual voice even in this giant room filled with all these other voices. I can't believe that my little unborn child recognized the sound of its father's voice. I can understand the auditory reasoning behind it, but this concept of personal acknowledgement is so much grander. *How can you know my voice?* I thought, looking at Lori's bump. *How can you separate my voice from all of the different noises you are hearing? You are still so little, yet you know your daddy?*

My friends set up another wine tasting weekend and planned to head north to Traverse City in the final days of April. I knew it was quite close to the predicted date of the birth, May 5th. If Lori went into delivery early, I could hop in my car and speed there in two hours. And considering my lifelong desire to tell a cop my speeding was due to the birth of my first child, it would really only be one hour and fifteen minutes. I asked her if I could go, and she was kind enough to agree.

I enjoyed the time I spent up north with my friends. We made a similar trip around the vineyards, even stopping for another toast at the exact same winery where I originally told them about my impending fatherhood back in October. Then we took off for dinner at the haunted Jolly Pumpkin Brewery on Old Mission Peninsula. We must have been such a pain to wait on. We didn't stop asking questions about the local restaurant ghost and finally got the details out of our waitress about what and where things happened, about which mirrors to look into and repeatedly say this or that. Then we all went back to the borrowed beach house Zac had acquired, ate more food, drank more booze, and played Cards Against Humanity.

The next morning, we were all milling about the house when Zac told me that the group had gotten together and purchased a present for me. I was in shock! They sat me down and explained how they knew the past few years had been rough for me, and with this new baby, the next few would be tough as well. But they told me I could always trust them to have my back as my eternal supporters. Then Marissa handed me a small black box. I opened it up to find a silver necklace with a small Latin engraving on it: *Flecti Non Frangi*. I looked beneath it and saw a small piece of paper with its meaning: "To Be Bent, But Not Broken." The paper also said that the engraved raven is a symbol of hope and is believed to have keen vision that pierces through all the darkness.

I looked up at my friends who were all huddled around me and smiling. There are no words to describe my gratitude for these people at this point in my life.

A few weeks later Bob Goff visited Grand Rapids to speak at a local church. I took Lori and our special package of an unborn baby in to see him. I love watching Bob speak. He's an emotional fireworks display with the ability to bring massive groups of people to tears with his crazy stories and bizarre, wonderful outlook on love and life. After he spoke, I shyly introduced him to Lori, fully knowing he would accept her but still quite embarrassed about this situation. Bob practically lunged at Lori and embraced her in a hug. The he got down on his knees, right in front of Lori's belly, and started delivering a speech to our new baby that he or she had the best parents in the world and would be so loved by us. The last thing he said to our baby was that Dad was on a rocket ship and now headed in a new and better direction. My goodness, Bob. I don't deserve this type of love from you, but you offer it so freely. What I would give to fully grasp his mindset, fully loving everyone through any situation.

Over the past few years, I had felt broken. I had felt left behind. And at times I still felt forgotten by my God. But then there are moments like this. Moments when you can get away and celebrate with your best friends, moments when Bob Goff, your secret mentor, shows he loves you through the craziest parts of your life, and Lori, this new person who has entered your life in the most meaningful ways, offers you unbounded, irreproachable, and never-ending love.

Starting in January, I began to fall deeply in love with Lori. And somehow, she managed to overlook the disclaimer of death that came with my heart. I realized she was exactly what I wanted and precisely what I needed. My ability to love her came incredibly naturally, and when I made the decision to truly open up my heart to her, I realized my love for her was different from anything I had ever felt before. It wasn't focused on who she could be or the things we could eventually do together. It was simply focused on who she is, right here and right now. I started to slowly realize that the more love I felt from her, even when I didn't deserve it, the safer I felt to give even more love back to her in return. And most of all, I loved her for beginning all of this wonderfulness by simply having a schoolgirl crush on me.

But again, those are simply words, filled with vowels and consonants to create nouns or adjectives used to describe her. But I still can't find the right combination of those things in my attempts to describe when she smiles at me from across a crowded room and my stomach starts flipping, or when she tells me she's proud of me and I get embarrassed by how much that fills up my soul, or at night in bed, when she rolls over to start scratching my back and I can feel her warm breath spreading across my skin. Maybe there are no words, even words in different languages, to describe these feelings. Maybe that's why these moments are so pure. They can't be stained by any of our weak languages.

Somehow, through all of this mess that had become my life, through being diagnosed with terminal cancer, through a miserable divorce, through our shared public shame, she was the one who saw past it all and promised me she'd love me forever. Even, she said to me with a smile, if I was bent or broken.

TWENTY-ONE
DUE DATE

"SHE HAD AN ORGASM WHILE GIVING BIRTH."

Lori and I didn't need to look at each other to know a smirk had shown up on both our faces. Lori had convinced me to attend this class and Lindsay, our instructor and Lori's close friend, was explaining stories of how, due to the miracle of HypnoBirthing, women could feel very little pain and, on occasion, "intense pleasure" during the birthing process.

Week after week we went, and she would teach us breathing exercises, thought patterns, ways to remove pain through specific types of touch, and showed us videos of people actually going through the birth process in peace. Lori and I were suspect, but neither of us wanted to leave our friend's class. In fact, Lori had the "great idea" to invite Lindsay to be her doula. Then Lori could fully show how quickly she forget everything she learned on the day when our child was born.

Lori was due on May 5th, but our midwife, Yolanda, told us the baby wouldn't show up till about the 15th. And sure enough, as the 5th passed, Lori kept thinking every little movement was a sign she was going into labor. Each time I'd go into a slight panic, grab our birth kit, start changing the sheets, get water for the bedside, and so on. But at about 1:00 p.m. on the 14th, Lori started to express these feelings again. It wasn't until about 3:00 p.m. when I actually started to believe her.

Yolanda showed up around 5:00 p.m. carrying a birthing bag that included who knows what. I definitely saw a red canister of oxygen, which I chose not to mention to Lori. Yolanda did an immediate exam that showed Lori's cervix was at six centimeters, meaning she was officially in labor. So, Lori called Lindsay, who showed up around 8:00 p.m. And as the sun went down, clouds started moving in over Grand Rapids, with rolling thunder shaking our windows and lighting setting the mood for an evening that was, no doubt, going to be intense.

Lori started to get nervous, unsure of the amount of pain that was to come. She moved around the house, lying on the ground, doing lunges, rolling on a yoga ball, sitting on the toilet, all while being reminded to take deep breaths. She threw up twice in the bucket she carried with her. I reminded her, as I had been telling her for weeks before that moment, that I would be right next to her no matter what happened.

Knowing I was going to be in the middle of this, I shouldn't have been surprised that during one of her contractions, she leaned over and, in agony, bit my shoulder. I did a silent yell as she half-heartedly apologized mid-contraction, but then later, she bit my hand. While I was sitting there rubbing my hand, I started to remember the stories from our class where women would actually break her man's hand by squeezing it too tightly. Fearing this, I would slowly start to suggest other options outside of hand holding, for instance, I could massage her neck or rub her back.

We were previously told a moment will arrive where she will want to give up, that she'll admit she can't handle it and try to quit. We were told that was the hump we had to get past to know the end was near. And sure enough, it came. I have never seen such pain. She looked at me with tears in her eyes, and said, "David, I can't do this. I don't want to do this anymore. I feel like I'm dying." I focused in on her eyes and reminded her of her days as a marathon runner and how we discussed beforehand that this moment, right now, would be so much harder. I just kept telling her she only had a few miles left, so just keep running because the finish line was in sight. I looked down and saw my necklace hanging outside my shirt. "Bent, but not broken." I considered bringing up that concept, but then I thought a woman in labor can only handle so many metaphors.

At midnight, Lori was fully dilated and Yolanda manually broke her water. That sped up the process to the point when Yolanda told me that I could see the baby's head. Yolanda pulled out a mirror and showed Lori the baby's head. Lori even reached down and felt it. That simple action gave Popeye her spinach. Lori, now knowing the end was close, was reinvigorated and moved from two mediocre pushes to five heavy pushes a minute, even breaking blood vessels in her eyes, face, and neck. Her entire head was becoming so dark red I actually started to get concerned this wasn't normal.

But the baby stayed there long enough that Yolanda started showing some concern. I could tell she was getting worried, so she finally increased her volume as she said, "Okay, Lori, this is it! Push Now! THE BABY HAS TO COME OUT ON THIS PUSH!"

What we didn't know at that time was that the baby had been stuck for so long it had stopped breathing. But Yolanda didn't tell us this mid-birth. The baby finally came out and Yolanda, knowing exactly what was going on, immediately began breathing into the baby's mouth to ventilate the lungs.

A few seconds passed until Yolanda saw that everything was fine. Lori and I were both desperate to know if it was a boy or girl, so I reached down to move the umbilical cord. It was a girl. Lori and I looked at each other with giant grins on our faces. Lori turned and with shortened breath said to Yolanda, "I know her name!" I turned and repeated Lori, "I know her name, too!" With our new baby girl in her arms, Lori said, "Hello Marian!"

Yolanda put Marian into Lori's arms and, after ensuring her that everything was okay, Lori attempted to feed her baby. After seeing Marian take to the nipple well, Yolanda left the room to go downstairs and begin her reports. I crawled onto the bed with what seemed like a never-ending smile as I cuddled up to Lori and our new baby girl, Marian. She was seven pounds and seven ounces and twenty-one inches long. Marian was gorgeous. I know all parents say that, but the photos of her just moments and even days after her birth, showed she was indeed absolutely perfect.

We named her Marian David Wenzel. At that time, we still had no idea how long I would be alive. I was just shy of five years into my five to seven-year sentence. Lori and I decided that no matter what happened, Marian would always know she was named after her father, whose name meant "Beloved," and that Marian would always know she was eternally loved by her earthly father, as well as her heavenly one.

This is my baby. This will one day be my girl. This will one day be a strong woman. Marian, our little surprise, is my flesh and blood, and yet here I am, facing down my own death. My heart ached at the thought of my unknown future. I now understand what T.S. Eliot meant when he wrote that "the purpose of literature is to turn blood into ink." But now all I want is for this ink to continue pumping through my heart, long enough to show her how to hold her breath underwater, teach her how to ride her bike, crash her first slumber party, attend her first play, scare the shit out of her first boyfriend, stand up and whistle as she walks across the graduation stage, and walk her down the aisle at her wedding. Marian, I so badly want this life to happen to both of us at the same time.

I have come to accept that living life is similar to writing stories. So, Marian, understand this book, this story I have written for you, was prompted by the words of author, Annie Dillard:

> *"One of the things I know about writing is this: spend it all, shoot it, play it, lose it, all, right away, every time. Do not hoard what seems good for a later place in the book or for another book; give it, give it all, give it now. The impulse to save something good for a better place later is the signal to spend it now. Something more will arise for later, something better. These things fill from behind, from beneath, like well water. Similarly, the impulse to keep to yourself what you have learned is not only shameful, it is destructive. Anything you do not give freely and abundantly becomes lost to you. You open your safe and find ashes."*

Oh, Marian. I don't know how much longer the story of my life will be. But I do know my single greatest regret would be lying in a hospital bed and cursing myself for not writing this book. For these words I kept in my safe for you to be discovered as ashes. For you to never understand the love I have for you. And to tell you that, above every other human, sermon, or book, you have taught me the most valuable lesson I have ever learned about God. Let me share that with you.

In the weeks and months following your birth I would hold you and you would cry. As babies do. But it became so intensely loud, I would try everything I could to get you to stop. I would sway you, I would pat your butt, I would "shh" your ears creating white noise. But your screams were so loud they were actually giving me intense headaches. I hate to admit I even got upset with you, squeezing you too hard, patting you too intensely, shushing you so loud it probably hurt your tiny little ears. All I wanted to do was drop you in your crib so that I could pass out in my own bed.

But one day it hit me. In the same way that you cried and screamed and moaned, completely unaware of me, a loving father who would do anything to protect you, to hold you, to care for you, to even die for you, I was doing the exact same thing with my God in heaven. I realized I wasn't seeing you the way my Father God sees me. To God, despite any of my accomplishments, purposes, films, books, relationships, or knowledge, I was still a simple infant in His arms. I am a child, incapable of knowing who is holding me, incapable of knowing how much my Father in heaven loves me, incapable of hearing His voice because of how loudly I'm screaming at the condition of my life. I even forget I am actually being held, forgetting the feeling of His arms wrapping me up and holding me to His chest, not knowing that He would do anything under the sun to protect me, to care for me, to even die for me. Marian, now when I hear you cry, I no longer get upset at you. I am reminded of how much I love you, because I am reminded of how much my God loves me.

The prophecies haven't stopped either. My medical doctors gave me my latest. They told me one of two things will happen. Either I will have a random, middle-of-the-day seizure and not wake up, or I will slowly fade, losing my ability to speak and understand words until I eventually exist in a fog. Not knowing which would be my end, I felt rushed to write a letter to Marian to be given to her upon my death or incapacitated state. It's a personal history of her, the somewhat late, yet eternal, love between her mother and I, the hopes I have for her future, and a few life lessons I've learned along the way.

Essentially, it's a compilation of Dad-isms I needed to document before I'm six feet under. Without giving away anything special I've created for Marian, I thought I would include a small portion of my letter, listing a few of the life lessons I've learned.

No matter what happens to me, there are a few pragmatic things to pass along. They may be right or wrong, but nevertheless, it's how I saw the world around me. I really don't know how God managed to deliver his commandments in ten short points, but since I openly admit to not being God, I see no point to best Him.

1. Love your mother. She will never ever stop loving you.

2. You will fail, but never become afraid of failure. It is the only thing that will truly teach you how to succeed.

3. Do not pursue expertise. Expertise is an overnight sprint that can be easily purchased or manufactured. Its end-goal is convincing others you are right and they are wrong. It wins the majority of social attention, popularity,

and money, yet truly affects very few lives. Pursue Authority. Authority is a marathon of experiences and feelings you earn from repeatedly failing. But oddly enough, I've found it impossible to gain authority without gaining expertise.

4. The English language has twenty-six letters that, through simple rearranging, are capable of declaring anything. Technology continues to change, but well-written words will always serve as its backbone. No matter your purpose, learn to represent yourself well through writing.

5. In relationships, medicine, health, spirituality, and just about anything, you will see opportunities to address symptoms or to address the core cause. Learn to trust your gut, and keep digging until you can address that core cause. When you find and address it, all symptoms, be they direct or referred, will disappear.

6. Don't let technology win. In the end, you will miss real conversations and real touch with real people.

7. I have read much more than the average person when it comes to healthy eating, but I can't replicate the simplicity of Michael Pollan's advice: "Eat food, not a lot, mainly vegetables."

8. One of the main priorities for your life is to discover your unique purpose. It truly doesn't matter how long it takes to show itself, but you will eventually uncover it. From this, the majority of life will follow, from relationships to financial priorities to the big decisions you must make. I truly believe that knowing and holding fast to your unique purpose, your personal calling, will be your most important personal gift to offer the world.

9. You can have things, but make sure they are good things, because stuff can be outdated, rust, break down, or go out of style. However, the memories you create with your friends and family by experiencing the world around you will never leave you. Pursue experiences.

10. I believe in God, His Son, and the Holy Spirit. At points in your life, I imagine you will love, hate, and be indifferent to that relationship. You will eventually learn you cannot control God, but you also can't completely write Him off. Your relationship with Him will exist inside a faith-based tension surrounded by questions or scenarios you may never know the answers to. But as long as you live in open communication with God,

admitting your frustrations while remaining open to hear His response of complete peace, you will survive just fine. This is the only way I've found to make any progress toward true shalom; peace with God, peace with myself, peace in my relationships, and peace in my circumstances.

11. Don't live to earn money. I know you most likely won't understand this until you attain wealth. My only hope is that you learn this lesson quickly so you can get past it. Make enough money to survive, then pursue what makes you happy.

12. Indifference is the ultimate enemy. It is the father of boredom and mother of mediocrity. Care about anything, but care about it with everything you have.

13. Don't drink cheap wine.

14. You are born in a time where technology makes every moment compete for public attention and approval. But I sense that in your future, the information you choose to keep private will become your source of personal wealth. Of course, you will have many moments to share, but I suggest you document images, memories, feelings, tastes, and smells for yourself (and maybe your lover or best friends). You need no one's approval to enjoy your life, so don't feel the need to ask for it.

15. When it comes to fashion, be both timely and timeless.

16. It is inevitable that things must get worse before they can get better. Learn to embrace the sheer terror and humility of walking backwards in your personal journey of detoxification. This is required of all of us before a new and better path can be discovered.

17. Visualize any loving relationship as a new world you are exploring. Remember where you have visited and look forward to tomorrow's adventures. But above all else, with as much energy as you can muster, learn to be with your lover right here and right now.

18. Life is too short to hold or fear grudges. No matter the offense, deal with your anger appropriately. Quickly forgive and/or quickly ask for forgiveness. Then, press on.

19. To honestly engage with this life, you must learn to jump in the deep end, then figure out how to swim.

20. As you begin to define your purpose, you will discover it consists of decisions that lead either to results or relationships. It's rarely so cut and dried, but you will see how these decisions eventually lean one way or the other. Choose relationships. Results may or may not achieve an end goal, but a relationship, even at the expense of results, is the best eternal investment you can make.

21. Marry your best friend. I mean, come on, seriously, trust me on this.

22. If you feel that things are going wrong, don't be afraid to talk openly with your mom. If for some reason you don't feel comfortable, talk with Aunt Heather. And should things go really, really wrong, call Bob Goff at 206-571-9798.

23. And finally, as best as you can, be humble, thankful, generous, polite, say your "pleases" and "thank yous," and only lie to another person when you smile and thank them for a gift you don't care for.

The first song Marian's tiny baby ears heard while lying on her parent's bed was, "The Moon Song."

I'm lying on the moon

My dear, I'll be there soon

It's a quiet and starry place

Times were swallowed up

In space, we're here, a million miles away

There's things I wish I knew

There's no thing I'd keep from you

It's a dark and shiny place

But with you, my dear, I'm safe

and we're a million miles away

We're lying on the moon

It's a perfect afternoon

Your shadow follows me all day

Making sure that I'm okay

and we're a million miles away

Lori and I continued to sing that song to her each night, over and over and over again. But as this tumor destroys my once very good memory, I lost the ability to remember those simple words. I quit trying to remember the actual lyrics and began to sing prayers for her through the melody of this song. I would make my way through as many verses as I could and offer up as many prayers that God gave me to sing. Marian, no one will ever know the strange, yet uniquely lovely moments you have brought into my life. Thank you, my love.

Marian, when I go, I promise I'll see you on the moon.

TWENTY-TWO
~~CANCER~~ SURVIVOR

AFTER THE FIVE-YEAR ANNIVERSARY OF MY DIAGNOSIS, I was now called a "cancer survivor." But it felt like that word "survivor" was so much bigger than just my cancer. I had gone through too many MRIs, sat through too many meetings with doctors telling me death is on my doorstep, argued far too much in my attempts to connect with Amy, and cried myself to sleep too many nights after impregnating Lori. I honestly feel like I barely made it through all of this alive. Yes, of course I'm glad to be a cancer survivor, but more so, I am glad to be a survivor of my life.

In order to celebrate my survival, we held a party. Lori, Marian, and I were the first to show up at the Sandy Point Beach House. And soon after, my sister and mother showed up. My family is filled with planners, so I knew they'd be there to make sure everything was going okay. We made sure the airstream trailer in the courtyard had enough drinks for whoever decided to show up. I was pacing. I'm always nervous about how my parties go, but this party was quite different.

I saw my friends start to show up and my stomach started to churn. Some of them from work. Some of them from church. Some of them from late-night dance parties at Rocky's. I limited myself to only one drink to lighten my nerves, while allowing me to be fully on point when delivering my speech. I brought the words I had recently written at The Hut to explain the joy I felt to still be alive. But before I spoke, I looked through the crowd to make eye contact with Lori, and saw my dear friend Rob was now holding Marian. Most likely my little sister tapped on something glass and everyone turned to see me with a mic. Here we go…

Today, June 7th, 2014, five years after passing out in a room of four hundred experts at a fancy hotel in San Francisco and being rushed to Stanford hospital where a series of tests were performed to tell me that I have an inoperable brain tumor and only five to seven years left to live, I am proud to say that I am officially deemed by the American Cancer Society to be a "Cancer Survivor." It is a proud day for me, my family and my friends, minus one slight little problem: I still have this pesky cancer growing in my head.

Now, there are four typical treatments for my type of brain tumor. The first includes full resection or brain surgery. The second is chemotherapy, and the third, radiation. And one final fourth option—the one doctors barely mention—"Choosing to Observe." It took me over a month to agonize over this decision, but after being prescribed chemo meds and being fitted for a radiation mask, I called my doctor on the eve of my first radiation treatment and told her I wanted to observe. She explained I was "choosing my own death" and that in five or six months, as the tumor grew, I would return and beg them to carry out the conventional procedures. But I knew in that moment that this was the right decision. And here I am, five years later, continuing to observe my tumor.

Of course, there are still small issues. Like many tumor patients, I suffer partial seizures every day that affect my ability to talk. At times I step outside of parties for a few minutes, letting a seizure pass. On another occasion, I made an entire group of my friends exit halfway through the movie, *Les Mis*. Other times, I've been sharing this story on stage and lost my ability to talk, smiling nervously and taking a few moments to pull my act together.

At times, I've passed out for nearly twelve hours, experiencing Global Temporary Amnesia or short-term memory loss, and woke up responding to questions of "Who's the president?" with the answer "some black guy." I've passed out from seizures in my favorite Grand Rapids restaurant, in an airplane lavatory 35,000 feet over the Atlantic Ocean, and while showering at the YMCA when my body fell to the no-doubt fungi covered floor. Rumor has it, I was convulsing naked on the ground while another naked man rushed over to hold my head steady. I'm so very thankful I have no memory of this event.

But these are the events that come with "Choosing to Observe." These are the events that each and every one of you have put up with over the past five years. Whether I quit talking mid-sentence, slurred my words, or practically fell over as my right side went limp, you have been there to hold me up, tell me I'm okay, that I was all right, that I wasn't alone. I can't think of a proper way to say "thank you" for taking this journey with me, but I'll make a small attempt…

First off, I want to thank Micah McLaughlin, my naturopath. It was his crazy idea to fight this cancer naturally. At first, I admit, I laughed in his face, but today, five years later, I have yet to regret this decision. Thank you, Micah. You are a dear friend in so many ways.

I would like to thank my ex-wife, Amy. She entered this battle against cancer by my side with as much, if not more, courage in the face of fear as I did. And while our marriage did not work out, I will be forever grateful for the role she played throughout an entire decade of my life. Wherever she is today, I truly hope she is well and experiences nothing but happiness for the rest of her days.

Thank you to Leslie, the oldest and most practical of my sisters. Five years ago, she pored over the same cancer books I did and told me, through tears, that she would finally start feeding her kids organic fruit and vegetables. THIS was a seriously huge deal for her.

Thank you to my older sister, Angie, who somehow managed to find the time to research my problems and diagnose me with hyponatremia from 729 miles away. Ever since that moment, over two years ago, I've had answers as to why I seize and can take immediate action to avoid it.

Thank you to my mom and my dad. They continue to support me in ways I can barely count. Knowing when to push on medical issues versus knowing when to simply talk about the weather. They provide me with extra dollars here or there, but mainly, I thank them for their fierce prayers on my behalf. They are the most dedicated and loving parents I could ever imagine. I am truly blessed by them.

Thank you to my younger sister Heather and her husband Michael. Honestly, I don't know how I would have survived my divorce had they not been living in Grand Rapids. At the end, when I gave up everything, both emotionally and physically, there was no question as to where I would go next. Their home was open and welcome to me. I see them as the apex of unconditional kindness and patience.

Thank you to Lori, who has somehow managed to fill a gaping hole in my life so perfectly well. My mother stated the other day that I ended up with the sweetest girl on the planet. I couldn't agree more. Lori, I love you so very much. You are my lover, my partner, and my best friend. I am reminded of this every time you tell me it doesn't matter how many days I have left, but that you will fully love me through each one of them. That is the best gift—well, maybe the second best gift you have ever offered me.

Speaking of the best gift, finally, thank you to Marian. Five years is a lot of time for heartache. I hate to admit that the majority of my hope was wrung out of me and I came to a point where I had nearly given up on life. I would never have killed myself—I'm far too vain for that—but I just stopped caring about everything. I became indifferent. But, Marian, then you showed up. And before you did anything, before you cried your first cry, wet your first diaper, or smiled that toothless, dimpled Wenzel grin, I am entirely certain that you saved my life by reintroducing me to hope. The nearly unbelievable story of your existence is my most-cherished story to tell.

So, cheers to every person who has entered this battle with cancer, no matter the final outcome. Each and every one of them are survivors, no matter how many years have passed. Cheers to Marilyn Amstutz, David Reiber, David Kuh, Matt Chandler, Adam Foster, Sarah Thebarge, Margaret Feinburg, Christy Ferebee, Daisy Merrick, Mille Juarez, Great Aunt Aldeena, Grandmother Ethel, and my Granny Louise. All of you serve as such an inspiration to me.

Cheers to a Holy God who, despite our best efforts, typically ending in complete and utter failure, continues to show us mercy each and every morning, turning our cancers, our divorces, and our surprise pregnancies into some of the most thrilling stories we could ever imagine. Today, five years later, I have a new home, a new love, and a new precious daughter. The life that cancer intended to destroy was saved by a God capable of turning my messy life into this celebration of goodness.

Cheers to "Choosing to Observe" love. To entirely forgetting the conventional ways of day-to-day life and choosing the alternative. To looking your friends in the eyes, observing their being, and telling them to their face how much you adore them—that your existence would be so shallow without the depth of their love. I hope we can choose to observe this wonderful life filled with so much love.

Cheers to "Peace and Love." Cheers to Ed Dobson who taught me to seek True Shalom by finding complete and utter peace with God, with ourselves, with others, and with our circumstances. And cheers to Bob Goff for displaying love the way Jesus intended us to see it. Let us all know that God truly is in control, and despite our fears that He isn't, let my story show you that our Lord will fight for you by bringing you, despite what you think is best, to discover True Shalom and true love.

Cheers to this present moment, right now on this beautiful Saturday in Michigan, surrounded by so many incredible friends and family. Cancer, I've got five years on you, but every additional moment I am offered, be it one more decade, one more year, one more day, or even one more breath, I will count each of them as a gift. And someday my time will come, and I will die, but I will die the happiest of all men, full of gratitude for the nine thrilling lives I have been blessed with.

But until then...

Cheers to this cake. Similar to my brain tumor, it's partially filled with chicken wire. (Kidding!) This celebratory cake, whose mere existence simultaneously represents both the worst and the best news of my life. It represents that yes, I still have cancer, but it also represents a moment for us to officially celebrate this day when I declare myself a cancer survivor!

In a time-honored tradition, only performed on my cancerversary, we all gather around you, carrot cake, and out of sheer and utmost respect, we salute you with the bird as I blow out each of your five candles. Cancer, you may soon strike my heel, but in time I will crush your head. Cancer...you sentient son of a bitch, we claim this moment for the living!

As promised, we set out a perfect cake, lit with candles for each and every June 7th that had passed since my diagnosis. It was strange to those who were celebrating this with me for the first time, and I can only imagine how it looked to the restaurant we were at. But I had everyone flick off the cake as I blew out the five candles. It felt strange to have just given that speech. To know I was living, breathing, loving. To know I am still alive.

Next, I walked directly towards Lori to give her a hug before she shooed me away to go talk to others. But strangely enough, no one approached me or came up to talk to me. Maybe they were too nervous, so I just kind of stood there alone, half in awe of what I just declared and half in concern over what I just declared. Finally, Caton, who noticed me standing by myself, came over and lowered his head, raised his eyebrows, and asked if I was doing okay.

"Yeah," I replied.

He asked, "Do you need anything?"

I didn't know what I needed, but then I grinned.

"Whisky."

Without saying another word, Caton took off to grab it.

"Wait!" I yelled as Caton spun around. I took a look at Lori, smiling as I saw my beautiful girl in the middle of another conversation across the party.

"Maker's Mark whisky," I said.

He got it.

I always say the best prayers when I've had a few drinks. Maybe I'm sitting on our front porch swing having a beer or in the middle of a giant crowd on the dance floor. With no more conscious self to edit, I offer pure and honest thoughts before my God (which is really all He ever asked from us in the first place). Maybe this is why Jesus asked us to have communion with wine, to get us all to relax, to take deep breaths, reminding us our daddy is holding each of us close to Him. That He hasn't left us. That He hasn't forgotten us. That He is willing to do anything for us, even die. Just so we can know He is willing to take us through the shit of the wilderness to bring us to our Promised Land.

I looked around me at this event. Everyone there had played such an important role in my life. I had this new woman who deeply loves me. I had this beautiful child. I was surrounded by a group of friends, even my darling mother who had cried and prayed for me. What else could I ask for? I was so glad to be there, with all of these people. Alive, breathing, and slightly tipsy.

I feel I have created so many good things with my life. But I also know I have destroyed so many things as well. But I didn't destroy with the same intent as God. I destroyed because of my selfishness, my greed, my vanity, my need to avoid permanent bonds. But then I thought through all of God's creations for me, my miraculous moments with people I never had a chance to thank. The nurse who, before my surgery, had read about my story on Jasmine's blog. Andy Cass who, due to a simple phone call from Don, volunteered his time to pick up a complete stranger at the Minneapolis airport. And the Wilsons who placed that same stranger to sleep in their Minnesota home. The gentleman I met in North Carolina who, during our trip to dinner, walked up to me and said, "Hey buddy, God is going to take care of you. You're going to be healed." I told him thank you for walking this tough road with me and that I appreciated his thoughts regarding my cancer. "Cancer?" he said. "Oh, I didn't know anything about that. God just told me to tell you that you'll be fine." I thought about the naked man who crouched over me and held my head as my naked body convulsed in the shower at the YMCA, and how he returned to my locker (fully toweled) and made sure I was okay. I thought about Dr. Fan's wife, about Tom, Steven, and Dr. Smeltzer, who all gave me the exact same prophecy that something incredible, better than birthday presents yet still unknown to me, was on my near horizon. I knew nothing of any of that at the time, but it turned out to be my Lori and my Marian. My new life and my new family are my "N/A."

People have asked me if I would ever want to get rid of the cancer, to restore my marriage, to not have knocked up Lori. I always, without a second thought, say "No." Because now I know I desperately needed that emptiness in my life in order to know how full my life is now. I had to see the bare, broken down forest before I could appreciate all of the new and beautiful trees around me. And I can nearly guarantee you, if you asked anyone who has suffered, they will always choose to never give it back. They hold that suffering so close to their heart because those were the moments they discovered who they were. Those were the moments when they held on tightly to those around them. Those were the moments when tears and anger and joy and peace actually meant something to them. Those were the moments when they turned to stare down God and eventually, like Job, put their hand over their mouth, having no more words to offer. They would never give up on those moments of suffering, and neither will I.

I have always said, I'd never believe in a God who didn't give me a Jesus. But now, I think I can confidently say that I'd never believe in Jesus if I didn't have you. Yes, you, reading this right now. You're bent, you're messed up, you're barely hanging on. But you, yes, you, the cheaters, the refugees, the drunks, the teachers, the sick, the small-town preachers, the volunteers, the sorrowful, the prisoners, those with stories publishers would never fund, and creators of music no label would promote: you are so perfect to me. Because of what God has both given and taken from each one of you, you have become my Jamaa. You have become my eternal family.

So please, for the love of God, you must keep going. Don't stop with me. When you visit others in situations similar to mine, those diagnosed with cancer, those struggling with horrible mistakes, give them yourselves. Give them your hope by hugging them like Micah. Offer them your peace just as Ed taught us. Shower them with love, like Bob did, by quietly sneaking away to do their dishes, then love them loudly by hiring a biplane to leave a smoke signal of a giant heart in the sky above their home. Please, don't let your religion ruin your love; don't become a Pharisee. Silently and graciously give to your lover, give to the needy, give to the sick, give to the poor in spirit. It's you. God has offered you for those in need around you. I can honestly say that your impact on my life is what makes me believe there is a Jesus, and Jesus is what makes me believe there is a God. I am overwhelmed by you, and I am overwhelmed by those of you who have given me this gift of telling my story. And now I know *"we'll meet again, don't know where, don't know when. But I know we'll meet again some sunny day."*

But the craziest of all is you, Lori. Let's forget our taxes, empty a bottle of Maker's Mark, split a *torta de jamón*, listen to Pink Rabbits on repeat, and skinny dip in Lake Michigan. Let's move to Iceland for a month, pop champagne, and rewatch every episode of *Breaking Bad*. Let's give ourselves permission to become the people we were born to be. Let's lean into the dark and help pull the sun up without falling asleep. Let's raise curious kids and never get tired of answering their question of "why? why? why?" Let's be surprised when it's our turn to die, realizing we accomplished everything we truly cared about.

There have been many great poets, yet none so great as the one who composed you. He describes through your eyes and rhymes through your lips. And when I read your poem, my love grows for you. I've waited, cried, laughed, kissed, turned from, ran toward, wooed, cursed, and somehow, I've stumbled on this wonderful mystery known as you. I grin, knowing full well it was better for us to sing the Beach Boys in beautiful harmony than reading the Scriptures in hateful discord. Feel the corners of my lips as they curl upward and listen to my beating chest as I breathe you in. You were my unknown buoy in the middle of my deepest and darkest waters; so, take your time, look hard, analyze each second, and please know my gaze is fixed on you. Lori, look at me and know that I love you.

TWENTY-THREE
BOLÉRO

MY FATHER HAD A PIECE OF MUSIC STUCK IN HIS HEAD: *SCHEHERAZADE*. You'd know the melody if you heard it, and I heard it over and over. When we'd work in the garage, he would loudly whistle this melody to himself as an unconscious expression of pleasure that he was enjoying his task. He always told me he needed my help, but I never actually did anything except sweep up after he was done. As I grew, I realized that maybe he just didn't want to be alone in the garage. But to this day, his song is yet to change.

And I am my father's son, which means I have a piece of music stuck in my head as well: *Boléro*, by Maurice Ravel, a piece I didn't care for when I first heard it as a child. My father used to take my family to the Orpheum Theater in Omaha, Nebraska to *culture* us. And throughout my life this song keeps showing up. Each time I hear it, I'm faced with the decision of whether or not I actually like it. But it wasn't until recently, when NPR's *RadioLab* did a podcast entitled, "Unraveling *Boléro*," that my interest was piqued. But first, the performance of *Boléro* …

Maurice Ravel was a very well-known French composer who wrote a number of brilliant pieces. In the late 1920s, he began working with Claude Debussy, creating a new movement called Impressionism. This music was very flowery and dreamlike, sensual, with lots of colors. In 1928, Maurice was commissioned by ballet dancer, Ida Rubinstein, to create a new song for her upcoming performance. Ravel dilly-dallied while writing this piece. But on his holiday in St. Jean-de-Luz, Ravel, who was about to go swimming in his pink bathing suit, swoops over to the piano, takes his index finger, and played the entire melody of *Boléro* to his friend Gustave Samazeuilh. "Don't you think this theme has an insistent quality?" he asked Samazeuilh. "I'm going to try and repeat it a number of times without any development, gradually increasing the orchestra as best I can." And he did.

He decided not to make this composition flowery, as was his style at the time, but to simply repeat the melody again and again. The theme doesn't change one note, but bit by bit, the orchestration grows, as the music continues to crescendo as instruments are added around this central and repetitive melody. For 340 bars, it never changes. While Ravel was finalizing the piece, the dance routine was being created by Rubinstein. This piece was composed for a ballet, and those attending the event would need a small hint about what would be happening on stage. So, they printed the following in the program for this premiere, telling the audience what they would be seeing:

> *"Inside a tavern in Spain, people dance beneath the brass lamp hung from the ceiling. In response to the cheers to join in, the female dancer has leapt onto the long table and her steps become more and more animated."*

Everyone in town was excited about Ida Rubenstien and Maurice Ravel's new collaboration. But Maurice, being a harsh critic of his own work, felt differently. While he was still actually writing the piece, he said it had "no form, properly speaking, no development, and no or almost no modulation." In 1931, a few years later, in a newspaper interview with the *Daily Telegraph*, he spoke about the work: *"It constitutes an experiment in a very special and limited direction, and should not be suspected of aiming at achieving anything different from, or anything more than, it actually does achieve. Before its first performance, I issued a warning to the effect that what I had written was a piece lasting seventeen minutes and consisting wholly of 'orchestral tissue without music'—of one very long, gradual crescendo. There are no contrasts, and practically no invention except the plan and the manner of execution."*

The composer of this song admitted his own music was quite ordinary.

On top of his dismal prediction of what was to come, he didn't really care for Ida's dance moves. At that time, he said his preferred stage design would be in an open-air setting, in front of a factory, which would reflect the mechanical nature of the music. Just imagine what the program would say for Maurice's version of the piece: *"Outside a widget factory in France, a group of people in tuxedos and monocles escort their French ladies in fancy Parisian dress to listen to music that sounds like machines. Due to their shocked responses, everyone gets drunk, starts a riot, and burns down the factory."*

It gets better. On November 22nd, at the premier of *Boléro* at the Paris Opera, a woman in the audience is reported to have stood up, mid-song, and declared that Ravel "had gone mad" as she turned and ran out of the room. Later, when told of this occurrence, Ravel smiled and remarked that she must have actually understood the piece.

How can this be? How can this same *ordinary* song be seen one way by Rubenstein, the ballet dancer, as a thrilling opportunity to jump up on the table and dance, also be seen as *ordinary* by Ravel, its composer, and set in a factory where everyone is silent and standing in long lines creating widgets? For years afterwards, people would argue about the tempo, speeding the melody up or slowing it down. Everyone had their own opinion on how this music should be played. But still, it was all the same *ordinary* music.

To some, it's brilliant, over-the-top Tits and Ass. And to others, it's maddening, simply This and That. Same song. Different reviews. Same notes. Different opinions.

But interestingly enough, and unknown to Maurice Ravel, this composition was born out of a sickness in his brain. He was at the height of his career when he composed *Boléro*. But six years later, he began forgetting his words. One night, he grabbed the wrong end of a knife and unknowingly attempted to cut into his dinner with the knife's handle. Next, he visited his friend for a chat, then forgetting his visit, returned two hours later and brought up the same issues. In 1935, Ravel's language skills were starting to evaporate. His personal journals still exist showing him practicing the alphabet, writing "B" over and over again, desperately wanting to relearn his letters.

Decades later, an American scientist, Anne Adams was doing cancer research, developing cancer cell lines that still exist and are used today. In 1986, her third son got into a horrible car accident. She was told he'd never walk again. But Anne, while at home taking care of her son, decided she wanted to quit science and become a painter. (Luckily enough, her son did learn to walk again, but Anne's life was changed forever.) Only a few days after making this decision to stay home, she had converted a room into her studio and began painting houses, buildings, and churches. Then she started painting intensely colored versions of cells and bacteria. Next, she moved onto painting strawberries. Water faucets with strawberries, planets made from strawberries, strawberries swirling around the universe. She completed images focused on strawberries thirty-four times. She would work all day long as her paintings got bigger and bigger. For someone who had not painted since high school, her work had become prolific.

In 1984, she decided to do a painting representing Maurice Ravel's *Boléro*, which she had become obsessed with. She began playing it on the piano, then started mapping out the piece, giving each note a color. Then she began another massive painting, a blizzard of triangles and symbols representing certain aspects of the piece. Little rectangles march along with triangles on the bottom of the picture, whose height represented the increasing loudness of that verse. The piece was becoming a representation of musical language. In this painting, her art replays Ravel's desire to repeat itself over and over again. But then in the second panel, as the music comes to an end, things unravel, hence *RadioLab*'s name for their podcast, "Unraveling *Boléro*."

But somewhere below the surface of Anne's creative mind, there was something else going on.

In the beginning she had absolutely no idea who Maurice Ravel was, and she named this piece without knowing of his life, or of his death. This is bizarre because Ravel's previous mental issues were now starting to show up in Anne's life. In 2000, Anne started to forget words just as Ravel did. She would try desperately to find those words, but couldn't. Anne ended up visiting the University of California in San Francisco. In 2002, they gave her tests that were videotaped showing Anne composed and sitting at a table. She looks as though she would know the answer to any question asked of her, but she doesn't. She can't remember which state she lives in, her town, or even her home address. Her ability to recall has completely been lost. When she would look at an image, she could barely manage to name what she was seeing. "Dog, star, watch." She was extremely frustrated. Both Anne and Maurice's minds were unraveling in the same way, sixty years apart.

Boléro, in both cases, served as the first symptom of their disease: Frontotemporal Dementia. This disease operates in a patient with primary progressive aphasia, a degenerative disease of the human language network. However, it also expresses another element: emergent transmodal creativity. It begins when this front-left portion of your brain starts to wither and die. Anne's brain scans show this happening, and the same is suspected of Maurice, despite the lack of brain imaging at that time. Before Ravel died in 1938, his doctor opened up his brain and saw the frontal left portion of his brain was disintegrating. This was the part of the brain that accomplishes many things, like storing memories, recalling moments, finding proper words, and the formation of language.

Eventually, both Anne and Maurice lost the ability to access this language portion of the brain. And when this happens, it changes how the brain works, enriching other parts of the brain, offering overwhelming sensations, causing patients to understand how beautiful this world truly is. Many patients with this specific disease start pursuing art with an insatiable need to create. Doctors say this creativity is based on a simple mechanical malfunction. They get stuck in an obsessive loop, like Ravel's *Boléro* or Anne Adams' paintings of strawberries.

This symptom of obsessive repetition begins early on in the course of this illness. And this desire to create may be driven by a condition that won't be seen for another six years. But as that prefrontal portion of the brain starts to fade away, the need for repetition starts to take over. So, these patients begin to create art that is obsessive and repetitive, yet beautiful and abstract.

This disease is extremely rare. And while I am dealing with some of its early symptoms and my tumor exists in the exact same portions of my brain, affecting similar functions, the chance of this exact disease occurring in me is nearly impossible. But *Boléro*, the same annoying music my father forced on me as a child, has returned to become my favorite classical piece, my "fight song." I listen to it frequently, using it to push me forward, using it to continue creating for as long as I am able. But over time, the doctors tell me my long-term memory, my speech comprehension, and my instant recall will continue to fade. I know I have already lost so many words and names, and those close to me say they can see it in my everyday life. All I can do is pray it's not the onset of Frontotemporal Dementia.

This morning's breakfast is remembered the same way as last week's breakfast. I can't remember watching movies. Sometimes after making a suggestion, Lori pleasantly reminds me I've already seen that one. Each morning I lay in bed trying to remember what we did last night. I can't remember simple children's songs, like "The Moon Song." I can read through magazine articles over and over, each time feeling like they're new to me. I will begin asking a question and halfway through forget what I was talking about, pausing, and asking what I had just said. I don't remember what I wore yesterday, so now I'm starting to downsize my wardrobe to make it easier: seven days, seven shirts.

So many people preach the words, "Live for now!" or "Be present!" It's not nearly as exciting as they make it out to be. Lori, my dear sweet Lori, recently purchased a small framed card for me. It sits next to me in my office and says, "Run the mile you are in." It's the only thing that has saved me of late. It's so easy to be overwhelmed by everything going on around me, small noises, repetitive drips from water faucets, small cries from the room over, tiny snores, shopping lists, directions. Everything is fading and I am currently struggling, learning how to handle this slow, yet ongoing deterioration of who I am. It seems my life is downsizing to a single moment in time, a single repetitive verse, continuing over and over again until the day I die. It's easy to become overwhelmed by all of this, but this is who I am right now. I am *Boléro*.

At the core of our human experience, I believe we all face one decision: *How will we handle right now?* Some of us will live without much hope, depressed, thinking everything is meaningless and empty. While others will declare this life to be thick with meaning and full of rich experiences. I know I can't speak clearly for everyone, so I'll speak to the group to which I belong: the Millennials, the white bread, middle class, suburban Americans. C'mon, you know who you are.

To my Millennial generation: We won't be poor in our innovations. We won't be poor in our adventures. We won't be poor in fulfilling our dreams. But we are and will be poor in our spirits. Despite everything we have been given, we are the loneliest generation because we put our dancing-together-on-the-table relationships behind our repetitive, factory-based 1s and 0s. We currently, and knowingly, are sacrificing what makes us human, and I hate to inform you, but there are no virtual realities, no holograms, no artificial intelligences, no self-driving cars, and no social media imprints to replace the meaning of what we will soon lose.

We were created for God and we were created for each other, but it seems our desires to make our lives easier, faster, and stronger are only making our lives worse. But I am positive that right now, and in our near futures, we can grasp those opportunities to right this wrong, to see our generation differently, to eat dinner with silent phones stacked in the middle of the table, to no longer prostitute ourselves for a thumbs up or unintentionally harm each other in order to gather more "likes," and to start loving each other.

Friends, let us prophesy to one another with "I believe" cookies and "hang in there" lasagnas. Let us provide hope for each other to overcome all of our pain and suffering. I know many of us feel we are living in the valley of dry bones, but it's up to us if we want to see the love, misery, faith, death, mystery, forgiveness, or sadness of this life. Because it is *this* pain and this struggle that shows us our trip to the promised land always begins in the wilderness. It is in *this* pain and in *this* struggle where we can see our seemingly perfect Kinfolk and Peter-Pan lives are completely meaningless on this side of eternity. Only now have I learned that in order to be made great, you first must be made lowly. Only now have I learned that in order to be made whole, you first must be made bent (but not broken).

Let us never forget our dark nights that are daily overcome by the light of our rising sun. Let us never forget that every mess can still be turned back into order. Let us never forget that feeling of heartache, knowing that true love still exists. Let us never forget the snores in the middle of the night (as annoying as they may be), showing us we aren't sleeping alone. And let us never forget our crying babies, many of them never even planned, who remind us we have a loving Father God currently holding us so tightly to his chest, promising to never leave us, to never turn his back on us, to even die for us. *These* are the things that show us, no matter how annoying or frustrating they are, that we are not alone and will never live this life by ourselves. We have been given each other to practice our earthly capers on in order to properly prepare us for an eternity of loving each other in heaven.

Because of Ed Dobson, I know my cure has already been wrapped up like a gift for me. And I look forward to tearing off that wrapping paper one day, be it during this life or after. I am aware that the time I've been given to pursue love and peace on this earth, to display grace, mercy, and forgiveness is so very limited. So, I choose to follow my Teacher, my Carpenter, my Fisherman, the Son of David, and Prince of Peace. I choose to follow my Jesus, an authority and not an expert, who himself, admitted His own miraculous earthly cures were never the end all, but pointed people toward eternal healing and living in True Shalom with God.

To those of you who are struggling, know there is no shame in calling out those struggles when they show up. Don't deny them. Don't hide from them. Gather your army and face them together. Knowing you have eternal victory over them, stand up and look them squarely in the eyes. Because *those* are the struggles God has allowed into your existence, offering you the chance to live a deeper and richer life. Try seeing your next struggle, be it your job, your relationship, or your finances, as just another repeating verse in your *Boléro*. And as your version presses on at your own constant tempo, make sure you keep turning your volume up, because as your laughs echo, as your tears flow, as your victories are won, and as your struggles are lost, you are slowly but surely becoming a beacon to this world. What will your beacon say? I pray our voices will together declare the love for our true Jamaa, our eternal family led by Jesus Christ and our loving God.

If you are still with me, you must get loud about your love. Hug each other. Don't update your status. Laugh with each other. Don't tweet. Cry with each other. Don't Instagram. Love one another. Because one day, like the last seconds of *Boléro*, when the music crashes in its final moments, our dance will end. And in that moment, your only desire will be bowing before your God who has been watching from the audience, as He rises to give you a standing ovation, welcoming you into His glorious heaven and declaring He is proud to be your God.

Now you have an opportunity to make this decision for yourself. You could choose to view your life as a factory, stamping widgets as Maurice knowingly composed his masterpiece, or you could choose to jump up on that table, throw back some wine, and dance your ass off with your bent-but-not-broken friends. Because, as you now know, you have limited time left; quite possibly five to seven years.

So, let's join together and declare in unity the benediction words used every Sunday by Reverend Chandler Stokes at Westminster Presbyterian Church:

Let's go into the world in peace, have courage, hold on to all that is good, never return evil for evil, strengthen the fainthearted, support the weak, help the suffering, and honor all people. Love and serve the Lord rejoicing, through the power of the Holy Spirit that makes each step possible. And may the grace of our Lord Jesus Christ, the love of God, and the sweet communion of the Holy Spirit, be with us now and forever more. Let the people say:

Amen.

EPILOGUE
I AM STILL ALIVE

"WILL YOU MARRY ME?" I asked. We had brought Marian to Fredrick Meijer Gardens and were sitting on my "thinking spot" in the tropical conservatory. It was November, and with temperatures dropping, we wanted to take a few minutes in the conservatory to remind us of this past summer with our new baby now sitting in Lori's arms. I presented Lori with my Granny's wedding ring that my mother had recently snuck to me. And then my dad gave Lori his father's wedding ring for me, with our initials etched in next to my grandparent's initials. Maybe we were a little too excited about our growing love for each other, considering I had gotten Lori pregnant again. We both knew we wanted more siblings for Marian, but this came rather quickly. Considering the only time we can get our families together was the holidays, we decided to get married on the day after Christmas, one month later.

In early December, we were visiting Ryan and Jenny Duffy for dinner, and after arriving at their home I was feeling pretty horrible. I went and lay down on the floor of their son's room. But that was the last thing I remember. I had another massive seizure. They called the ambulance which rushed me off to a downtown hospital. I kept having more seizures, so to stop it they had to keep me unconscious, which means they had to intubate me. And every time they tried to wake me I'd try to rip the tube out of my throat. Avoiding the potential hazard of damaging my vocal chords, they chose to keep me unconscious for a full week.

When they finally woke me up, I learned what had happened. The last thing I remember was being at the Duffy's house, but now an entire week has passed. After coming back to consciousness, I was trying to sleep and experienced unbelievable pain behind my right knee. It is somewhat strange to say, but that may have been the most extreme amount of pain I've ever experienced. They told me I had a blood clot behind my right knee and needed me to stay in the hospital for another week.

I got out of the hospital on Christmas Eve. Then we celebrated Christmas (of which I remember absolutely nothing) and then Lori and I were married the next day. Given the fact we had absolutely no money, we decided we would get married in The Sparrows. That was the closest thing to a home that Lori and I had. Plus, it had enough space to fit our 50–ish number of family members and a few extremely close friends.

Heather was my "Best Wo-man" and Todd was Lori's "wo-Man of Honor." We had a lovely ceremony held by Tom Sprague, a dear friend I had met at the Vineyard Church. I whispered my way through our vows due to my one-week stint with a massive tube down my throat, which caused me to lose my voice. Then we went to a party space downtown and celebrated with all of our friends. Heather and Michael had purchased us a night at the JW Marriott, the fanciest hotel in town. But unfortunately, I was so tired from my two weeks in the hospital and entertaining at the wedding and reception that I couldn't perform my husbandly duties.

After all of the excitement from our wedding, we ended up going back to Mayo where we met with my doctor regarding my recent major seizure. After looking at my brain scan, he told me that he was quite convinced I would not see my next daughter born and should begin to prepare my family for that. He practically begged me to take part in conventional treatment, even saying that if I didn't, Mayo would no longer see me as a patient. Again, to hear my doctor tell me I'm about to die scared me, but I refused to believe him. I continued repeating to myself, *I am still alive.*

After returning home from Minnesota, Don Miller called us up to say he was speaking in town. Lori and I met with him at Reserve, a lovely restaurant downtown where we shared dinner. After hearing about my recent seizure news, he told me that his mom had gone through Proton Therapy radiation and was feeling much better. In addition, he said that Scott Hamilton, the Olympic gold medal figure skater and friend of his, was convinced this was the best treatment possible and was currently raising money to build a proton therapy treatment facility in Tennessee. In fact, there are only nine locations that perform this procedure in the United States. After lots of prayer regarding going back on my initial agreement to fight this cancer alternatively, we decided to go in for treatment.

Lori and I took Marian on her first plane ride, and we went to stay with my sister Angie and her husband, Jamin, in Moorestown, New Jersey, across the river from Philadelphia. The plan was for me to receive a six-week course of Proton Radiation at the Abramson Cancer Center through the University of Pennsylvania's Penn Medical Center.

During my time in therapy I was unable to drive due to my previous seizure, even though my sister had a spare car sitting in their driveway. I jokingly tried to convince her that because I was in a different state, the rules didn't matter. She didn't bite. So, Angie or Jamin would take me to their local train station, then I would take a thirty-minute ride into the city, then walk about a mile and a half to the hospital. The weather was miserable and I was freezing because I didn't think I'd need my winter coat. I probably lost weight because I wasn't drinking alcohol and was walking nearly four miles a day.

Unfortunately, during my time there I ended up losing things. I lost my weekend duffle bag filled with my favorite clothes: my APC jeans that had been perfectly worn in over the past five years, my favorite jacket, my perfect pink Gant t-shirt, and my new APC sweatshirt that I bought the day before for too much money to keep me warm in Philadelphia's early spring. I also lost half of my hair; literally split down the middle of my head due to the radiation. I also lost my daughter's name. One night while journaling, I went to write her name and couldn't remember it. Instead of looking it up or texting my wife, I sat there and forced myself to remember it. I thought and thought, but the only thing I could remember is that is started with an M. It was a half hour filled with curse words and tears before my lovely daughter's name came back to me: Marian.

Every radiation session, at the same time, when the position of the beams was facing that same specific portion of my brain, I could smell my skin burning. Each time I smelled this I became ridiculously depressed, feeling as though I had turned my back on my alternative healing plan. I had moved from treating my body as my fighter to now relying on a $250 million machine that cost me $500,000 to use. Those six weeks were rough. I returned home with a half a head of hair, half of the clothes I brought, and a collection of burned memories.

Right when I returned home, I knew I wanted to start going to church again, but this time I wanted Lori by my side, because after all, she did start believing in God again. So, we started attending Westminster Presbyterian Church where Heather was on staff. And as though Reverend Chandler Stokes knew I would be there that morning, he preached on how the church should be the most hospitable place on the planet. It was a salve after being away from church for so long. However, at the end of my time in Philadelphia I had purchased a top hat to provide coverage for my half-head of hair. And sure enough, on that first Sunday, after hearing a lovely message about how everyone is welcome at this church, I had an old woman come up to me and screech, "In MY day, we didn't wear hats to church." Goodness gracious, I was literally waiting for someone to make a comment about my half head of hair so I could unleash the hounds of hell on them, but if I truly unleashed on this woman she probably would have fallen over from a heart attack. I was extremely pissed as I took off my hat and told her through clenched teeth that the radiation for my brain cancer caused me to lose half of my hair. Then I just stared her down. The look of surprise on her face was priceless.

Viola Madeline, our second daughter, arrived on May 15th, 2015. One full year and one full hour after Marian was born. They are truly Irish Twins. She was named after my Great Aunt Viola because they all share the same birthday. If she wasn't born on Great Aunt Viola's birthday, she would have been named Daisy, after my Granny who died of cancer in 1989.

It turns out that Viola was born with a set of lungs. She was the loudest baby we had ever heard. In fact, we had two separate daycare workers tell us that she is the loudest baby they had ever heard. Having added another infant with our one-year-old was quite difficult. But over time we realized Viola, or Wawa as Marian called her, was our reckless one. Always scratching her skin while wildly flailing about, slamming herself into stationary objects, failing over again and again. Her body still looks as though we beat her.

But after a little more time, we saw she was always injuring herself or breaking the rules to help others. Anytime we needed to discipline her, we realized she was doing something for someone else. She would steal a toy from Marian, but then present it to Lori. She would be digging through the dog food bowl and we'd raise our voice to tell her to get her hands out, and she would turn around and innocently offer us the piece of trash that had fallen into it. She would struggle to open the front door and we would yell that she shouldn't be walking in the front yard, and then Cali would walk through the door and give her a little lick on the hand. Looks like our reckless monster is simply a monster of love.

Ed Dobson died of ALS on our one-year anniversary in 2015, but I am certain he died in peace. Then, a few months later, Bob Goff's Malibu lodge burned to the ground. In 2008, when Dot&Cross went to the lodge, it became a tradition that everyone would climb underneath Bob's long kitchen table and sign their names. And after eight years of signatures from amazing people, I can only assume the smoke from those burning names under the table created a smell so sweet to our Lord above, like a beautiful sacrifice of love and creativity. I suppose that's a pretty great reason to go back again with my whole family one day and sign the bottom of the next table again.

My neighbor, Johnny Clauson, and I went and performed a Viking funeral for every item I ever received from Amy. I had a pile of cards, trinkets, wedding photos, and a DVD of our engagement we promised we wouldn't watch until our ten-year anniversary. I suppose firing arrows at this stuff is just as crazy as when she burned our books and movies in her brother's backyard. However, I felt like this experience had a little more flair.

Johnny and I found fallen trees, chopped them up, and fashioned our own raft with twine. We secured all of our items and tied a rope to bring it back just in case something went wrong. We practiced with his professional bow before we lit our arrows dipped in jet fuel. And as we began to shoot, the first few were slightly off target due the drag of the lit rags on the front of the arrows. Understandable. But when we started getting closer to lighting the raft on fire, the speed of the arrows would blow out the flames in mid-air. Eventually, I was shooting from a log (mainly because it was the best potential for a great photo) and ended up losing my balance and falling into the dirty and leech-filled water. And no, it wasn't a glorious fall, more like a cartoon fall with my legs and arms flying in all directions while smacking myself in the head with my bow.

Nevertheless, I still wanted all this stuff burned, so I waded out into the water and tossed a lit arrow on top our hand built funeral vessel. It didn't end up being the glorious flaming fire I had always seen in movies, but in the end, it worked. After getting out of the lake, I took a piss toward our flaming vessel, then we sat together, threw back a few more All-Day IPAs from Founder's Brewery, and watched as my past relationship burned and sank.

Next came our third girl, Henrietta Jane, born on August 30th, 2016. Having three girls under three years old intensified our crazy lives even more. The move from a man-to-man defense to a zone defense was nearly overwhelming for Lori and me. Crying was happening and no one could explain why. Scratches were being distributed with no reasoning. We were overcome by messy diapers. And our only savior at mealtimes was our dog Cali, who would come and eat up all the food thrown on the floor. At the end of a long day, when Lori and I practically fell onto the couch in exhaustion, we would be ripped away from our relaxation when a toy, night after night, randomly blared out music from "Old Macdonald." We finally figured out that as the sun was setting it would trigger this toy to play. We thought it was our living children haunting us after they went to sleep.

But to be honest, I think that's all I care to say about our children. Because if you have kids, you are absolutely positive *your* kids are the cutest and the smartest and the worst and the messiest. So, it does me no good to claim those things for my own children. And if you don't have kids, you have absolutely no idea what I'm taking about anyway and none of this makes any sense to you. But if you're lucky, maybe one day you'll find out.

In December of 2016 I went to see Dr. David Bertram, a doctor in Neuroscience at Spectrum Health. I signed up for the exact same test I took when I moved into my condo after Amy and I split up in 2011. Dr. Bertram reminded me that my IQ doesn't change, but in some of the tests, changes in my IQ can be measured. He took me through the whole process again, reminding me that the brain still has the same capacity to remember, but the issue is measuring the processing and encoding of new memories.

I did all of the same tests I did at Pine Rest, the hand grips still proving my left hand is stronger than my right, drawing a clock then drawing a specific time on that clock, connecting dots with the corresponding letter (A, 1, B, 2, C, 3). They measured my level of general intelligence by asking questions that are a little harder each time. But I realized they had new random questions. I was feeling good about how many questions I got right, but my mind blanked when they asked me who wrote Sherlock Holmes. *AHH, Come on! You know this David!* I only had so much time to answer and somehow blurted out William Conan Doyle, as opposed to Arthur Conan Doyle. But he determined I was close enough to pass on that question, so he continued and I answered a few more.

After my tests, he sat me down and told me something I hated to hear. It wasn't that my brain was deteriorating (which he did say it was), or that my creativity was lacking (which he also said). He looked me in the eyes and told me, "I'm surprised you're still alive." What a gut punch. Anyone with any type of medical degree has told me again and again how surprised they are that I am still alive. I felt that no one else gets this. Everyone else feels I'm just dreaming up this diagnosis and seeking sympathy from others, but the doctors are treating me like I'm a miracle. I actually went home feeling anger and cried hot tears when I told Lori how upset I was that the doctor had told me this. It feels as though I'm living two different lives.

I've been on a continual path to learn how not to be afraid of the end of my life. But as Johnny Cash once said, "God gives us life and takes it away as He sees fit." I think that's about as simple as he could make it after living his long life filled with both pain and glory, so I'll accept his answer as my own. You can choose to make that quote as complicated or as simple as you want, but I'm sticking with this: *My life belongs to God. He gives and He takes. So, I'll just shut my mouth.* End of line.

Eventually, Lori and I moved from our rented home on Richard Terrace to our new purchased home on Holmdene Boulevard. Moving reminded me of when Lori moved into Richard Terrace. I remembered that the only thing left in the house was a tiny bottle of holy water sitting on the ledge above the front door. So, when we officially moved into our new home I surprised Lori and pulled out that same bottle of holy water and we put it on top of our new front door. That same night, when our girls were asleep in a room full of boxes and pack-n-plays, we were too exhausted to do anything. Technically we had everything in the house, but we had no idea where anything was. Lori and I offered a cheers to our new home as we drank a wonderful cabernet sauvignon. I drank my share from Etta's baby bottle and Lori drank straight from the bottle. Welcome home, Wenzels.

Our new home is lovely. It has a full lot on the side where our dog and our growing kids can go nuts. It's the topic of many of our conversations regarding sizes of trampolines, gardening strategies, potential yurts, small living spaces for my parents, potential future weddings, and so on. On our first day there, our neighbor approached us and said he was a retired cop and was now running a gun safety course if we were interested. So yeah, I would say our house is in a pretty good location. We have a Jewish Temple and a Catholic university one block south of us. A Christian Church one block east of us. A dog park a few blocks west of us. And a child rehabilitation center one block north of us is. Oh, not to mention VanderMill Cider a block north of us, an establishment we look forward to visiting at the end of our long summer walks.

And now here I am, seemingly completing the full circle of my unknown time on this planet. I live in a small city, in a suburb filled with pleasant people, in a home with my incredible wife and three children whom I desperately love. We drive a minivan. We attend church every Sunday. I mow the grass in my yard. I water our plants. I shovel the snow on our sidewalk. I own a dust-buster. I pick up my dog's poop. I empty my cat's litter box. (In fact, I'm responsible for six out of seven members of my family's excrement. Yup, 85 percent.) I am not what I imagined myself to be as a child or what I imagined myself to be in my twenties. But now, with special thanks to God, I am approaching ordinariness. No, it's not a "Tits and Ass" life, but it's also not a "This and That" life. I am now living a life marked by "Love and Peace," and I plan on living this life for as long as I can.

Lori allowed me to attend a weekend retreat by Lake Michigan. Kent Dobson, Ed Dobson's son, was leading ten men, each who were there for their own reasons. During one of our final sessions Kent told us to go out into the wilderness and communicate with God. I chose to walk toward the beautiful sandy beach, with the cool wind blowing through my hair so I could watch the last glimpses of the sunset while I thought back over the past years of my crazy life. And as I stepped onto the beach, it reminded me that Jesus told his followers to never build their homes on sand, as beautiful as it may be. But Jesus told all of us to build our homes on the rock. I suppose that means there's nothing wrong with existing at rock bottom while you start your life over again. It seems that rock bottom is typically where God builds his strongest foundations.

Kent told us to draw a circle for us to "own" and put something we've found at the top of the circle to serve as a reminder, like our north star. I was searching for an item but couldn't find anything. But then I spotted a small stone in the middle of a rock pile that seemed to leap out at me. I imagined it to be about the same size of the stone David would have picked up before his battle with Goliath. The same size stone that challenged that beast who continually reminded David he is about to face his own death. The same size stone he placed in his sling, eyeing the beast who laughed at him, calling him a fool for trying to fight. The same size stone David was preparing to hurl at the beast who was holding up pieces of paper filled with statistics for types of brain cancer. The same size stone aimed at this beast's head as it mocked him by reminding him his brain is no longer what it used to be. Determining I would survive this beastly enemy I am facing, I picked up that stone and declared it my north star.

Kent asked me to step inside of this circle, place my north star item at the top, and verbally declare it was *my* circle. I could see how this moment was affecting me similar to my time in The Hut while writing my five-year survival speech. So, with a small grin, I looked to the moon and howled to my wolves. A great big howl for my mama wolf, and three short howls for my little wolf pups. After that, I took off my shoes and put my rock in the shallow water at the top of my circle.

Kent had also explained that we should indulge in our imaginations and accept those little ideas that keep popping into our heads without feeling dumb or silly. And as I stepped into the water, my toes feeling the water filling between them, my imagination exploded with the image of a massive pirate ship about 100 yards out into the water. On it, I could see those who had died of cancer lining the side of the ship and cheering me on. They were telling me not to stop, not to slow down, but to keep pressing forward through the wilderness with my eyes undimmed and my vigor unabated.

I stood there, fully confirming what God was telling me in this moment. It seems so simple, but I've never really wrapped my arms around it. In order for us to accept His divine mercy when the water surrounds us, warms our feet, and fills up our souls, we must also be willing to accept His divine justice when the water rushes away and leaves our souls feeling cold, naked, and alone.

The shimmering yet freezing cold water rushed up past my north star rock to surround my toes before it retreated back into Lake Michigan. *Breathe in.* It came up around my dirty heels again, deconstructing its previous sand dunes as it spread itself around my feet, before uneventfully drawing itself back into the frigid black depths. *Breathe out.* Up, around me, filling the spaces between my toes, then followed by the cold air as the water slides away. *Breathe in.* Water coming in, rhythmically, up to my ankles, covering my war weary and typically misplaced feet, then dissolving back toward an eternal lake with another side I cannot yet see. *Breathe out.*

I feel the warm water gathering around my feet as I remember my nearly perfect upbringing, being constantly supported and encouraged to press on. *Breathe in.* But then the water recedes as I learn I have a life-ending brain cancer that will soon destroy not only my creativity, my words, and my memories, but my life. *Breathe out.* Then I discover my story is truly "Set Apart," and begin sharing my God-given story as my soul is filled up with life-giving water. *Breathe in.* My water evaporates, just as Amy did when she parted ways with me and, as I heard, moved back to California, the place she always knew would be her true home. *Breathe out.* But then the water swells up to nearly cover me as Lori shows up to love me unconditionally and straighten out my bent life. *Breathe in.* The water sped away again when I was let go from two separate jobs this past year, each of them destroying my sense of self-worth. *Breathe out.* But water returns to flood me with joy each time I return to our new home, kiss my wife, and hug a few girls who think I'm the best daddy on the planet. As my struggles seem to continually surround and overtake me, I must recognize and know my Father will repeatedly bring this healing water back to me, either in this life or the next.

The monotony of this seemingly never-ending process of breathing in and breathing out, of water lapping together, then giving into its own waves is miserably boring, but it is also infinitely beautiful. Our God, who is capable of creating and destroying sinless trees that have stood for over one hundred years, can, in a few seconds, give and take, just like this water constantly lapping up around me, then rushing away as I stand on this beach. Because in the end, one of these waves will eventually sweep us away from that rugged beach and we'll be surrounded by that heavenly water for the rest of eternity. Let it be known that this work of creation and this work of destruction is the continuous work of our loving and peaceful God in heaven. *Breathe in. Breath out.*

And now, all I have left to say is, "Glory."

THANK YOU...

THIS BOOK IS DEDICATED TO MY LORI, my earthly trinity. You have given me three ridiculously cute and life changing girls; Marian David, Viola Madeline, and Henrietta Jane. You continue to blow my mind with your two running-marathons-while-pregnant legs. And for your single soul, that same soul who chased me down and refused to give up on me until I finally realized we were created perfectly for one another. Thank you. Thank you. Thank you.

To the Wenzel Family and all of its cohorts! I want you to know how much I love each and every one of you! You have been a true gift to me since I was born, and I have no doubt you'll be that same gift to me until the day I die. I cannot imagine a better family to spend this wonderful life with.

To the Slager family, all 694 of you! You are the biggest, hottest mess I've ever seen. But so what? You keep proving your awesomeness every single time we get together. Your family is the perfect polar opposite to mine which makes me love you even more. Here's to the Slager clan and the next generation of Slager-Fest!

Thank you to Ben Arment, who threatened to beat me up if I didn't offer this book via Kickstarter. You are my true brother and I love the shit out of you! Thank you to Jennifer Zamzow for guiding and protecting this story, while making incredible suggestions when I needed them the most. Thank you to Tyler Huckabee, my cornhusker brother from another mother, who knew exactly what I wanted to say before I could even turn on my computer. Thank you to Derek Baird! I can't believe we only met once (the day before my first seizure in San Francisco), yet you have stuck by my side ever since. I thank you for the birthday cards for our girls, your social connections you've passed along, and your ongoing care for my cancer scenario which has proved you as a great (although long-distance) sidekick. And thank you to Chris Ferebee: You are an amazing friend in these crazy times of publishing and no matter what happened or happens, your friendship is worth more than gold.

Thank you to my Kickstarter family! I'm still in awe over the support you offered me when I sent out the call for help. YOU helped me raise my family while I was working on this book for eight hours a day. I'm sorry it was released a little late and hope you can forgive me, but as is typical, I was struggling to make sure all of the bills were paid while I was in the editing process. Please share this book with those in your life who need to read it!

Thank you for the musical inspiration provided by Josh Ritter, Over The Rhine, Arcade Fire, Bahamas, The National, Andrew Bird, Future Islands, Brandi Carlile, Father John Misty, Sufjan Stevens, and, of course, Johnny Cash.

Thank you to Gorilla who breathed life into this book! From your incredible Kickstarter promotion of this book, to your large donation that made this book happen, I want to thank you for believing in me. Special shout out to Eric for your work to create a remarkable promotional film and to Scott for the hours you spent editing my white, pasty bald head. I have been in awe as I've watched Gorilla move forward with their commercials, their documentaries, and their full-length films. I am so impressed you are always willing to negotiate prices to pursue the right projects at the right times and for the right reasons. Gorilla, you make great media, but more than that, you are a great group of people. Thank you so much. Find them at: wearegorilla.co

Thank you to Mascot Books for finding me when it didn't look like I could find my own way! I loved working with your professional staff, namely Maria, Debbie, Kristin, and your discovery of Lorna, who apparently knows more about proper grammar than the rest of us combined. Your services have been impeccable, and I look forward to continuing to work with you in the future. Your dedication to communication, editing, and design have been a godsend to me. The publishing world is now the wild, wild west, but Mascot Books understands how to make things happen and happen quickly. I highly recommend other authors to consider working with them as you share your incredible stories! Find them at: mascotbooks.com

DAVID V. WENZEL

David V. Wenzel was born and grew up in Papillion, Nebraska, went to college at Cedarville University in Ohio, then hesitated a bit too long in Santa Monica, California. At twenty-three, he moved to Grand Rapids, Michigan, where he and his friends started Dot&Cross, a multimedia firm where they produced films, wrote books, and created websites for today's masterminds of business and spirituality.

After learning of his cancer diagnosis in 2009, David created a new company, RobinHood Ink., to assist in building the dreams of forward-thinking companies who are looking to set themselves apart in their market. In December of 2014, he was married to Lori, and they have somehow managed to create three girls, Marian, Viola, and Henrietta, within three years of each other.

In June of 2017, he outlived the seven-year prognosis for survival he was given by doctors. Due to his desire to press forward against this sentient bastard of a disease, he created Bent Not Broken, a nonprofit company focused on providing support, motivation, and hope to cancer survivors.

Currently, he manages RobinHood Ink., leads the Bent Not Broken gatherings, and shares his story of overcoming cancer at conferences, churches, and schools across the country.

www.davidvwenzel.com